Cooking with Judith

Comfort Foods Create WOW! Eating

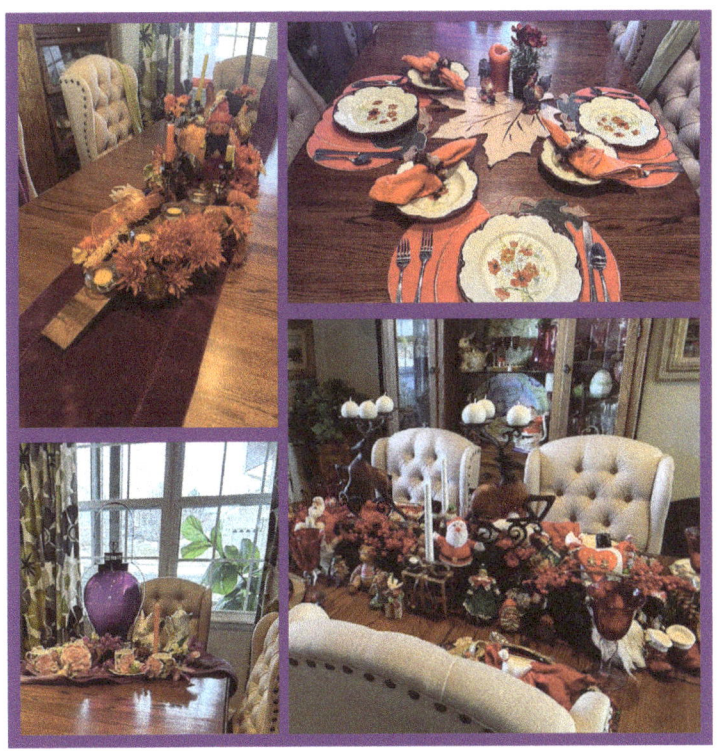

Dr. Judith Briles

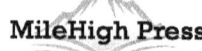

Mile High Press, Ltd.
www.MileHighPress.com
MileHighPress@aol.com
303-885-4460

**Cooking with Judith
Comfort Food can be WOW Food!**
Copyright © 2025 Judith Briles
All rights reserved.

DO NOT TRAIN
Created by Human Intelligence

No part of this book may be reproduced
in any written, electronic, recording, or photocopying form
without written permission of the publisher. The exception would be
in the case of brief quotations embodied in critical articles or reviews
and pages where permission is specifically granted by the publisher.

Although every precaution has been taken to verify the accuracy
of the information contained herein, the author and publisher assume
no responsibility for any errors or omissions. No liability is assumed for damages
that may result from the use of information contained within.

Books may be purchased in quantity by contacting
the publisher directly or by calling 303-885-2207.
Mile High Press, Ltd.
8122 South Quatar Circle
Aurora, Colorado 80016

Editing: Peggie Ireland
Cover and Interior Design: Rebecca Finkel, F+P Design, FPGD.com

ISBN trade paperback: 978-1-885331-99-1
ISBN eBook: 978-1-885331-12-0

LCCN: 2025901007

cooking | comfort food | entertaining

*Dedicated to

everyone I have

shared a meal with.

Thank you

for the good food

and great conversation.*

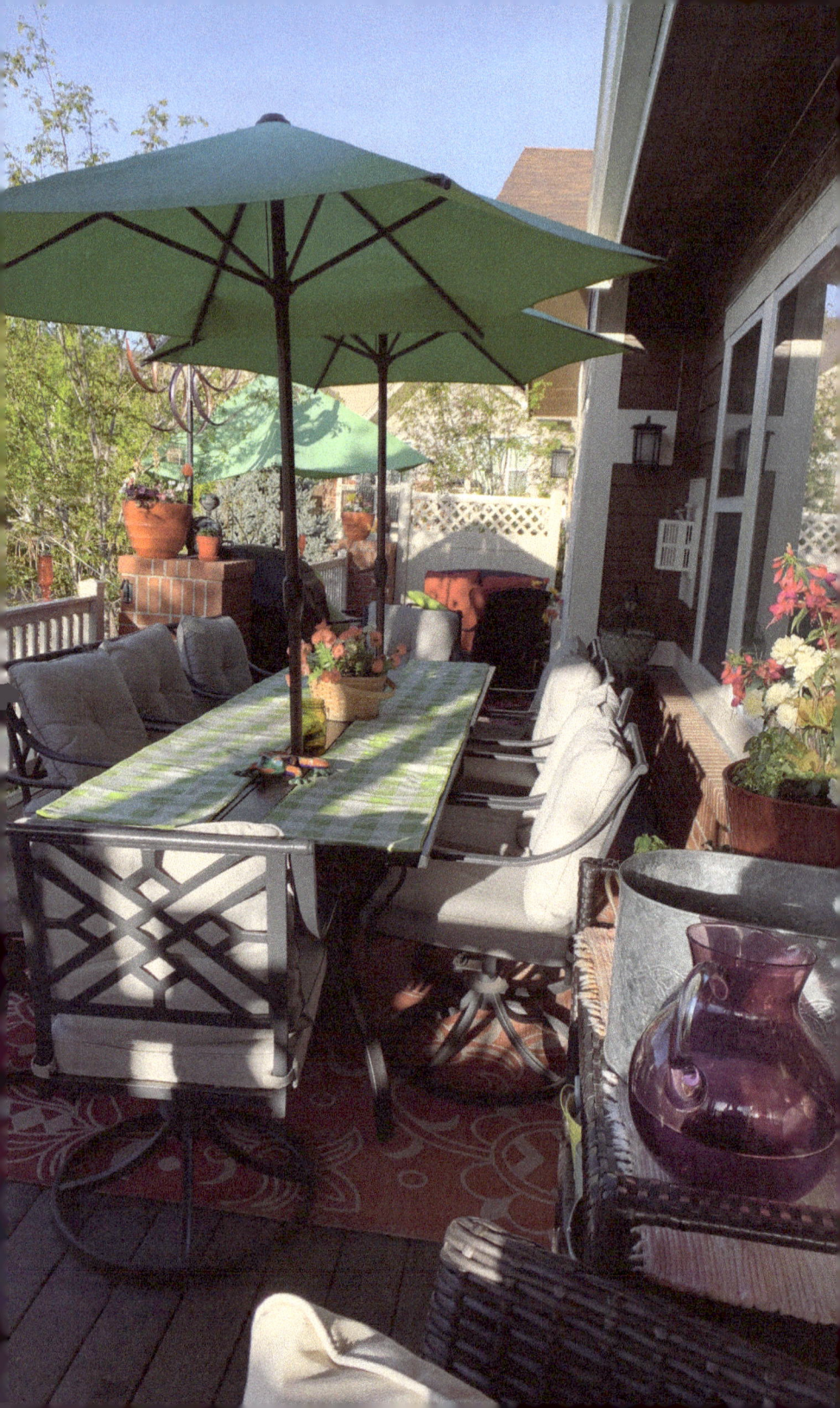

contents

Welcome to My Kitchen 9

appetizers

Bruschetta 11
Chicken Salad Boats 12
Judith's Bacon Smokies 14
Judith's Cheesy Crostini Bites 15
Judith's Fig Jam (or Marionberry),
Goat Cheese, Basil Crostini 16
Judith's Pine Nuts and Dates Crostini 17
Pumpkin Goat Cheese Crostini 18
Sweet Chili Cheesy Stuffed Mushrooms ... 19
Zucchini Patties 20

soup

Chioppino (aka Fisherman's Stew) 21
Corn Chowder Delight 24
Gazpacho 26
Judith's Chili Relleno Corn Chowder 28
Judith's Easy Peasy French Onion Soup 30
Pumpkin Soup 32
Red Pepper and Tomato Soup
with Croutons 33
Rustic Italian Tortellini Soup 35

salad

Avocado Corn Salad 37
Irresistible Grape Salad 38
Judith's 24-Hour Salad 39
Judith's Apple or Pear Pecan Salad

with Honey Mustard Dressing 40
Judith's Summer Beet Salad 42
Lobster Salad 43
Mardi Gras Salad 43
Pears and Pomegranates
Red Leaf Lettuce Salad 47
Red and Green Christmas Salad 48
Watermelon Salad with Feta
and Cucumber-Mint 50

sides

Asiago Bacon Capers and
Garlic Roasted Asparagus 51
Buttery Garlic Mushroom 52
Fingerlings 53
Mardi Gras Maque Choux 54
Orzo and Wild Rice 55
Pearl Onion and Cheese au Gratin 57
Slow-Cooker Creamed Corn 58

quiche

Judith's Muchroom Quiche 59
Quiche Lorraine 61

pasta

Creamy Corn Pasta with Basil
and Parmesan 63
Judith's Baked Spaghetti 65
Judith's Friday Night
Mexican Spaghetti Carbonara 67
Judith's Mac and Cheese 69

mexican

Chile Rellenos Casserole 71
Mexian Tortilla Festival 72
Taco Pie 74

seafood
Cod Fritters with Mango Salsa 75
Shrimp with Corn Salad 77

pork
Judith's Ham Steaks and
Cheesy Scalloped Potato Cheat 78
Judith's Pork Loin Medallions 80
Oktoberfest Pork Tenderloin 82

poultry
Chicken Swiss Cutlets with Avocados 83
Creamy Parmesan Chicken Cutlets 85
Judith's Plum-Glazed Cornish Hens 87

desserts
Chocolate Zucchini Cake 89
Judith's Baked Pears 91
Judith's Kahlua Cake 92
Tiramisu Made Easy 93

Essentials for Judith's Kitchen 95
　Pantry 96
　Baking ingredients 98
　Cooking 99
　Fridge 100
　Freezer 100

about Judith 103

*Inspired by one of my
favorite foodie quotes ...*

*A gourmet who thinks of calories
is like a tart who looks at her watch.*

— James Beard

Welcome to My Kitchen

'm not a chef or a gourmet, *but I am a cook*. I love the "presentation" and setting a table for the season or event. And I dabble and I play with combining foods, herbs, and spices. *Spoiler alert:* I never cook with thyme or rosemary, both I'm allergic to. All with the objective of tasty food and great tastes. If you came to my home for a cup of sugar, I may be able to help. If you were looking for a cup of capers, I'm your gal.

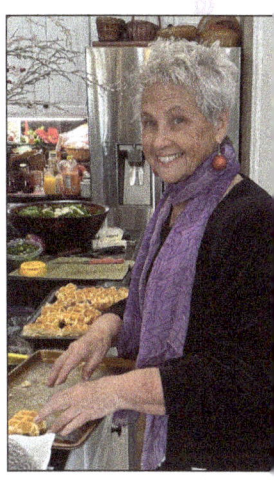

Sometimes I'll call a friend and share what I'm doing and ask if they would like to be my Guinea pig for a meal. No one turns me down. Some of my concoctions are roaring successes … some, well, I need to tweak a tad.

For years, friends, family, clients, staff, and visitors have asked me to share what I create. My truthiness is that I often just make things up as I go along, rarely making notes or writing them up. I'm a "hands-on" cook—meaning that I view other recipes as a starting point—I get to play with it. It means opening the pantry and seeing what talks to me. It means that I don't have to go to a specialty store for exotic ingredients. Hands-on also means that salads with greens are mixed with my hands—no bruising to the lettuce.

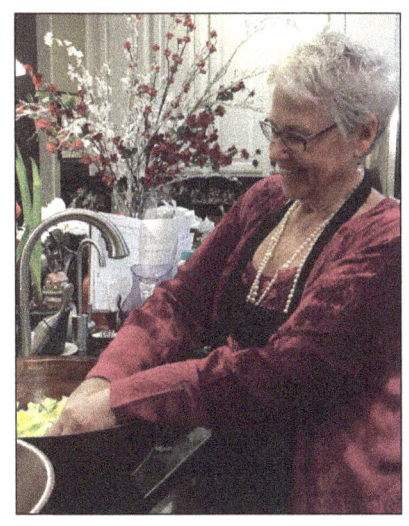

This past year, I started to make better notes and created files for recipes.

My intention was and is not to write a cookbook with an emphasis on entertaining around dishes. I didn't want to do that, although I love entertaining around food. With friends. Both inside and outside on the deck. I share randomly on my blogs and social media when I do.

What I have for you is a few of my dishes—appetizers, salads, main dishes and a few desserts—the Easy Peasy Tiramisu is always a hit. And my cheesy bite concoction is devoured as soon as it comes out of the oven.

Enjoy … and if you make any of them, share your photos with me. Make sure one of them has you in it and send to my email, Judith@Briles.com.

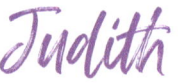

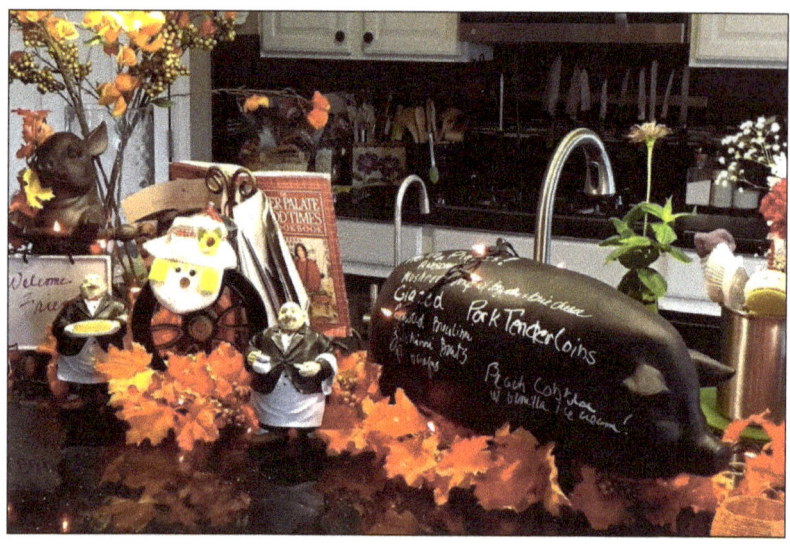

Bruschetta

A plate of bruschetta is often found on my entertainment menu. Sometimes they are simple and basic—like a diced tomato, garlic, and basil mix ... or with goat or feta cheese, soft cheeses, shrimp or veggies from the garden. They can easily be a theme: Italian, Mexican, Mediterranean, or Hawaiian.

They always start with a baguette that has been sliced, olive oiled and baked for a few minutes, cooled, then toppings added. When my back deck is opened sometime in April or May, baguettes are bought, sliced, olive-garlic oiled and baked. I keep bags of them frozen in my freezer for instant usage.

> baguette ... slice ½ inch thick. Olive oil or avocado oil mixed with garlic powder or garlic sauce to taste.
>
> Bake 5 to 7 minutes in 350° oven.
>
> add a spread—goat or a feta cheese
> *I love a Middle Eastern market where Hungarian, French fetas are readily available and taste delicious. Brie is also a favorite and, of course, pesto.*

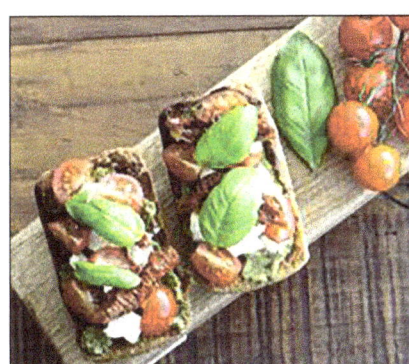

putting it all together
Now, what's your "add" combination? My go-to is chopped fresh tomato with pesto, garlic, and a kiss of balsamic vinegar. Think of a theme. Mexican would include chiles and tomatoes—maybe a little Mexican or Queso cheese. If Italian ... you may want to have small meatball in a tomato mix. If Mediterranean, Kalamata olives could be cut in half with feta and a little tomato. I love Kalmatas!

- Sliced baguette pieces
- Spread or not to spread on top of slice ... your choice
- Maybe something to drizzle on top. Balsamic is my favorite.

Serve cold

Chicken Salad Boats

Think of my Chicken Salad Boats as a perfect appetizer or mini salads. Perfect for small and large gatherings. They make about 20 boats and are scooped up quickly. One of my guests asked if I had extras in my other refrigerator. "Why," I asked.

"I have a party to go to tonight and need to bring something. If you have any extras, I'll buy them from you," was her response. "If I did, how many do you want?"

Ten was her answer. "I will make them for you. I have the leaves and filling—it will take me less than 10 minutes ... and it will be a gift from me to you." So, I did—and her friends devoured in minutes.

Makes 20 boats
ingredients

   2 C cooked chicken, diced

   1 C mayonnaise

   3 T capers

   ½ C celery, diced

   1C red or green seedless grapes, sliced in quarters

   1 T dill

   salt and pepper to taste

   Baby romaine lettuce

   1–2 carrots, shredded

putting it all together

I use either a pre-roasted chicken and cut it up OR bake two chicken breasts and thighs each. Dice them up. Mix all other ingredients. Scoop into lettuce leaves. Top with carrots. I usually do this all a few hours before I plan on serving.

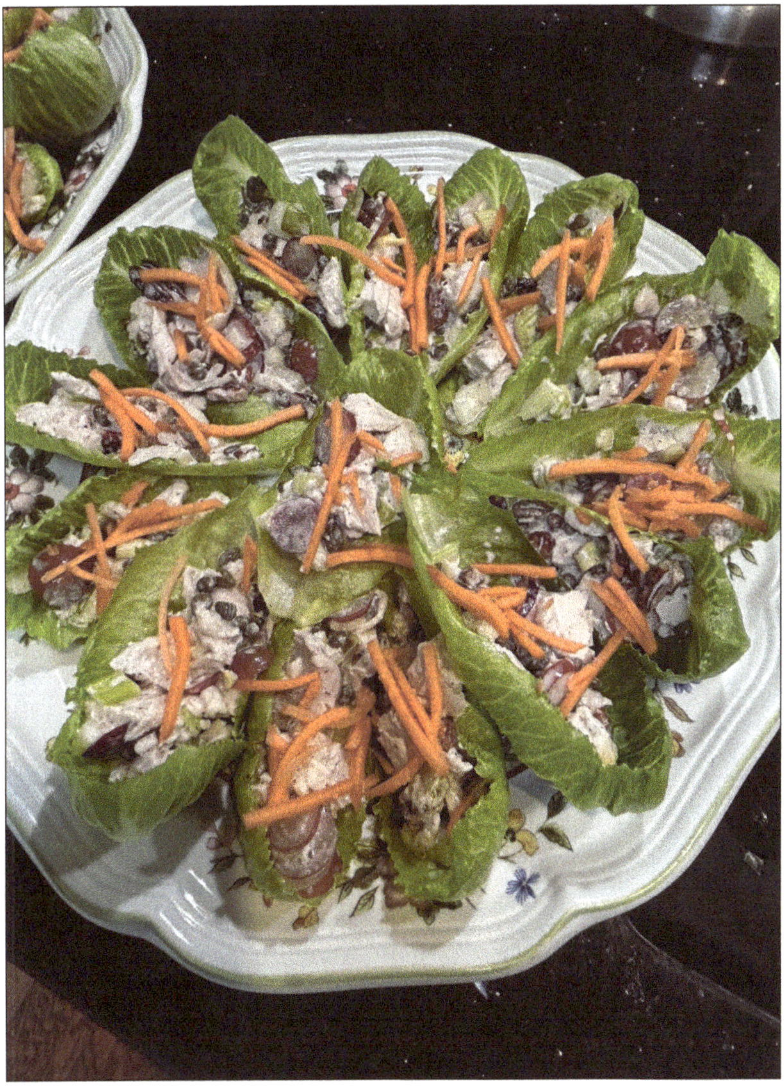

Easy Peasy Recipes That Are Quick and Delicious 13

JB's Bacon Smokies

We are an appetizer household. Sometimes appetizers are dinner. When I know I'll have a crowd, these bacon smokies are a favorite. Love it that they are easy peasy and I can prep a cookie sheet of them ahead of time. And I start cooking them 20 minutes before guests are expected.

Prep time: 20 min.
Oven time: up to 30 min. Preheat oven to 350°

ingredients

smokies, small bag, about 40 smokies

bacon, one pound

½ C brown sugar

maple syrup, enough to dissolve brown sugar and then cover smokies as you roll/dip them for the final bake.

Tajin seasoning–sprinkle in your mix … don't overdo unless you want "heat," but use for a spice.

putting it all together

Cut bacon strips into THIRDS. Wrap each smokie with bacon. Mix brown sugar, maple syrup, and Tajin. Roll smokies in sauce and secure with tooth pick.

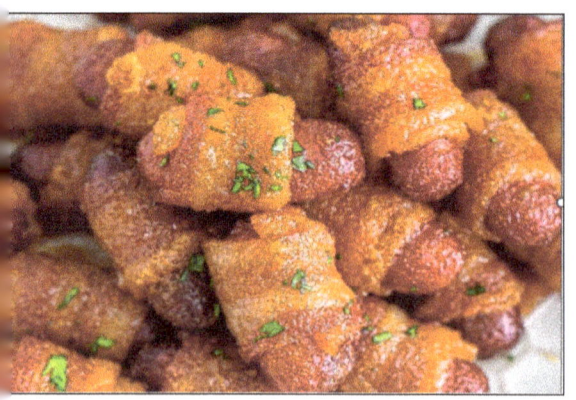

Bake for up to 30 minutes, until done on an foil lined cookie sheet until bacon is cooked.

Serve with or without toothpicks still in. They will disappear fast.

Judith's Cheesy Crostini Bites

ingredients

baguette, sliced – ½ inch thick … sourdough or white bread, crusts off (if you use this, you will cut into quarters) … or cocktail squared breads you can find in the deli section of grocery store.

2 T garlic, minced

¾ C Parmesan cheese, grated type, like for topping spaghetti

1 C mayonnaise

Preheat oven to 350°

putting it all together

In bowl, I add a large glob (don't hate me when I say this) of mayo, a few tablespoons of diced garlic and a bunch of Parmesan cheese and mix it all up. You want a thick consistency. So, for every cup of mayo, 2 T garlic, ¾ C of Parmesan. Adjust for taste and consistency. My crowd likes garlic.

Suggestion … I buy Costco's baguettes, at least two packages, each holding two large baguettes. As soon as I bring them home, I cut up one into ½ inch thick slices. This appetizer is rich so figure 2–3 pieces per person max.

Start watching your oven at 4 minutes. The crostini will harden a tad and the cheesy concoction will begin to bubble. A hint of browning is OK. Immediately out of oven, plate and serve.

Always devoured as soon as the plate is presented.

Judith's Fig Jam (or Marionberry), Goat Cheese, Basil Crostini

ingredients

> baguette – sliced and toasted in oven with olive oil and light sprinkle of garlic salt. *I do ahead of time.*
>
> jar of fig or marionberry jam *Marionberry is a personal fave!*
>
> goat cheese log
>
> basil

Preheat oven to 350°

putting it all together

Suggestion ... I buy Costco's baguettes, at least to packages that have two large baguettes in them. As soon as I bring them in from the car, they are cut up—typically two of them in four-inch pieces for pasta type dinners and frozen. The other two are cut into ½ inch thick slices.

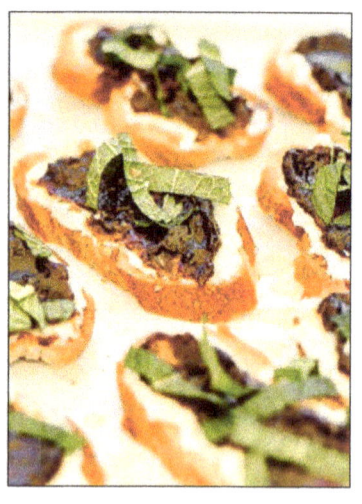

Add olive oil to a cookie sheet and garlic salt—don't overdo. Sometimes I add a little Parmesan to top each slice a minute before I pull out of the oven for cooling.

Start watching the oven at 3 minutes—whether you want a softness to each slice or more toasted is up to you. No more than 8 minutes.

Once crostini are cooled, **spread with goat cheese.** *Be generous.* Now, top with jam—at least ½ teaspoon—and either a full basil leaf or sprinkle a few chopped ones for topping.

Always devoured as soon as the plate is presented.

Judith's Pine Nuts & Dates Crostini

Yummy finger food appetizers are where crostinis enter your kitchen —just about anything that you can serve on a thin toasted bread ... bite size. My preference is always a baguette that is slice ¼ to ½ inch thick ... add olive oil, a little garlic salt and toast for a few minutes. I make ahead, freeze and always have them ready to add a dollop of my favorite spread, veggie mix of the moment and serve.

makes 12 crostini
ingredients

> ½ C pine nuts, toasted – 350° oven for about 8 minutes
>
> ⅓ C red wine, no preferred type
>
> ¼ C honey, or a tad more
>
> 6 Medjool dates
>
> baguette, sliced and toasted in oven with olive oil and light sprinkle of garlic salt. *I do ahead of time.*

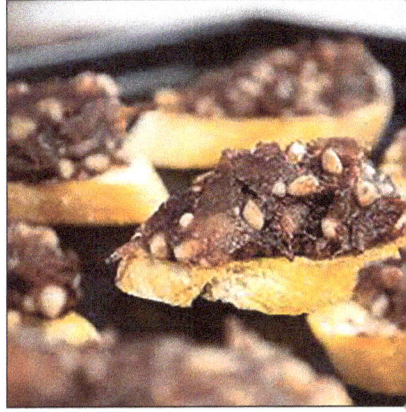

Suggestion ... I buy Costco's baguettes: two packages each holding two large baguettes. As soon as I bring them in the house, I cut up two baguettes into four-inch pieces for pasta type dinners and freeze them. The other two are cut into ½ inch thick slices. Preheat oven to 350°

Add olive oil and garlic salt to a cookie sheet. Don't overdue. Sometimes I add a little Parmesan to top each slice a minute before I pull them out of the oven.

Start watching you oven at 6 minutes. Time depends on whether you want slices soft or more toasted, but no more than 8 minutes.

Chop dates—add to stovetop pan: pine nuts, dates, honey and wine —cook down 3–5 minutes. Spread on toasted baguette—yummy.

Pumpkin Goat Cheese Crostini

It's the perfect intro into Fall time. I usually have a bag of pumpkin seeds in my pantry. My freezer usually has sliced baguettes ready to toast with a kiss of olive oil. And goat cheese is a staple in my refrigerator. Add fall spices—a little nutmeg or pumpkin pie spice, some maple syrup to your concoction and appetizers are minutes away.

Max time, including prep; less than 20 minutes.

ingredients

sourdough baguette cut into ½ inch slices and spread with 2 T olive oil.

putting it all together

Then mix following and add on slices prior to baking.

4 oz goat cheese, softened to room temperature

4 oz cream cheese, softened to room temperature

½ C plus 2 T pumpkin puree, canned or cooked

2 T pure maple syrup

½ tsp kosher salt

½ tsp black pepper

½ tsp ground cinnamon, nutmeg or pumpkin pie spice

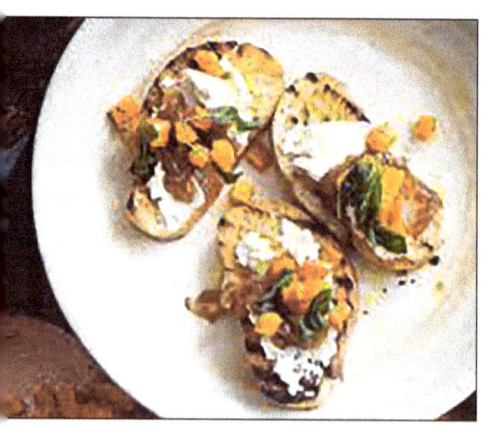

Final toppings when out of oven

3 T dried cranberries

2 T unsalted pumpkin seeds, toasted

Toasted crostini topped with a creamy pumpkin, goat cheese, and cream cheese spread is one of the best holiday appetizers!

Easy Peasy Recipes That Are Quick and Delicious

Sweet Chili Cheesy Stuffed Mushrooms

When I have friends over for dinner, I always have an appetizer. Whether it's hot or cold, appetizers are the opening number. Many times I have two: maybe a cheese selection or crostini with a topping that's appropriate for the season, and one of the easiest appetizers to whip up is a stuffed mushroom.

This one was a "concoction" that came together when I had extra Baby Bella mushrooms. My friend Kay was helping me prep for an event while my hand was in a cast. I pulled out cottage cheese, cheddar cheese, and Boursin cheese. Mixing them together, I added a kiss of garlic salt and reached for the Sweet Chili Sauce. Delicious.

Makes enough to stuff 30 mushrooms. Preheat oven to 350°

ingredients

Baby Bella, Cremini or White Oyster mushrooms—clean, remove stems. *Don't soak mushrooms, they will instantly absorb water. Rinse off and dry before stuffing.*

1 package of Boursin cheese. *I use herbs and chives.*

8 oz cottage cheese, regular or small curd

¾ C cheddar cheese

¼ C sweet chili cauce

garlic salt to taste

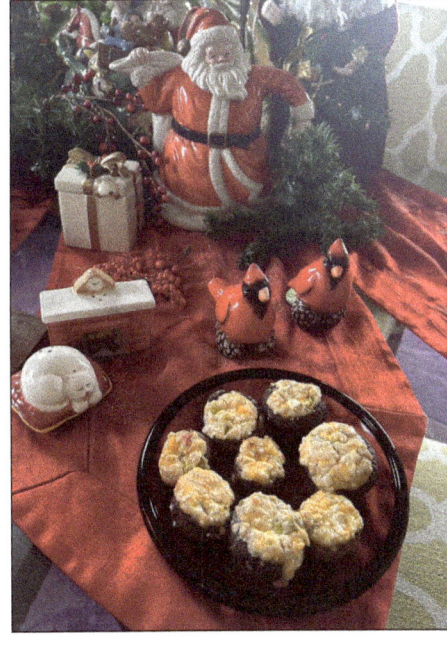

putting it all together

Mix all together and spoon generously into mushrooms. Place on cookie sheet or open baking dish. Place in oven and cook until mushrooms feel soft to touch—they are done.

Serve immediately.

Zucchini Patties

What to do with all the zucchini that summertime brings? This is the perfect recipe.

Side dish or a type of tapa. If you like a tad of spice, you can always add a bit of salsa in the mix. Trader Joes has a kick to it—or part of a seeded, diced Jalapeño. Makes about 8 patties.

ingredients

2 C grated zucchini, excess water removed …
I use colander, then paper towels.

½ to ¾ C freshly grated Parmesan cheese

1 C panko …
my two bits: panko is kickass to regular breadcrumbs

sprinkle of ground nutmeg, about ⅛ tsp … *Note:* If you add too much, it can quickly take over the taste; less is more here.

¼ tsp paprika

1 clove garlic, minced

2 eggs

½ tsp salt, plus more as desired

¼ tsp pepper

½ Jalapeño, seeded, if you want a little kick to it

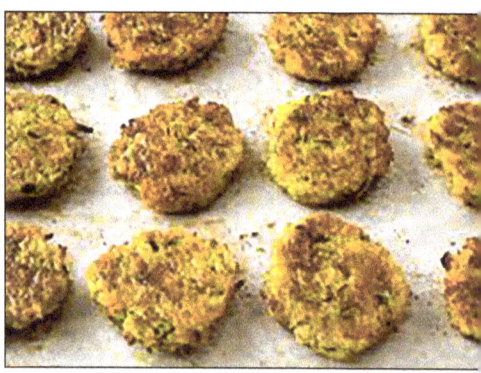

3 T avocado oil to cook in—add more if needed

putting it all together

Combine all ingredients, except avocado oil, in a bowl and mix thoroughly. Use a heaping tablespoon to form patties.

Heat oil in a frying pan over medium heat. Add patties and cook until golden brown, about 3-4 minutes per side. Serve warm.

Add a dollop of ranch dressing. *Enjoy!*

Chioppino (aka Fisherman's Stew)

I had my first delectable bowl of Chioppino at Scoma's Restaurant in San Franciso. With a salad and mouthwatering hot garlic bread for dipping, it was the ultimate complete meal for a seafood lover. John and I would drive the hour from our home ... then talk about how fabulous it was on the drive home.

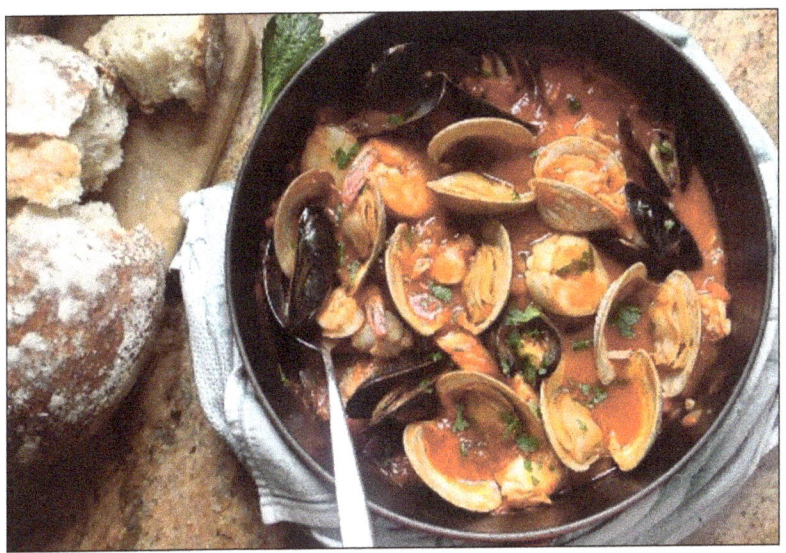

Now, I'll call a few friends for a causal dinner on the deck, lots of napkins on the table, and a deep dive into Italian heaven tastes amazing for seafood foodies with wine of course. I serve in oversize bowls with soup spoons—actually designed for chioppino—a large fish at the bottom is part of the design—natch!

Serves 10 to 12

ingredients

12 T extra-virgin olive oil, divided

1⅓ C finely chopped shallots, about 6-8 large shallots

6 cloves garlic, minced

2 C white wine

continued

2 (28 oz each) cans crushed tomatoes

4 (8 oz) bottles clam juice

4 tsp sugar

3 tsp salt, divided

1 tsp crushed red pepper flakes

1 tsp dried oregano

3 pounds firm-fleshed fish fillets, such as halibut, cod, mahi-mahi, salmon, or snapper, etc., cut into 2-3 inch pieces. *My preference is a firm white fish. I bake in the oven and place in soup bowl, adding the stew on top just before serving. The fish is firmer this way.*

6 T unsalted butter

3 pounds (about 18) littleneck clams, scrubbed

2 pounds mussels, scrubbed

1 pound scallops, cleaned—no sand welcomed

3 pounds extra-large raw shrimp, peeled and deveined

2 C water, may need more

Italian parsley, fresh, chopped, for garnish (optional)

dill for garnish (optional)

putting it all together

Preheat the oven to 400° and put an oven rack in the middle position. Line a baking sheet with aluminum foil and set aside.

In a large pot, heat 8 T of the oil over medium heat. Add the shallots and cook, stirring frequently, until soft and translucent, about 5 minutes. Add the garlic and cook, stirring constantly, for 1 minute more. Do not brown.

Add the wine and increase the heat to high. Boil until the wine is reduced by about half, 3 to 4 minutes.

Add the crushed tomatoes, clam juice, sugar, 1½ tsp of the salt, red pepper flakes, oregano, and 2 C of water. Bring to a boil; reduce the heat and simmer, covered, for 25 minutes.

While the stew is simmering, toss the fish with the remaining oil and sprinkle with salt or garlic salt. Cook about 10 minutes in oven. Cover and keep warm until ready to serve.

When the stew is done simmering, add butter. Add the clams, mussels, and bring the stew back to a simmer. Cover and cook until clams have mostly opened. Add shrimp and scallops, simmer. Remember, they cook fast to their pink, "I'm done" color. Cover and and cook until the shrimp are just cooked through and the clams and mussels are completely opened, about 5 minutes. Overcooking shrimp and scallops will make them rubbery and tasteless. Discard ALL unopened clams and mussels.

Now, divide the warm fish into the bottom of each serving bowl, then ladle the stew over the top, and take to the table.

Heated garlic bread for sopping is a must have.

Make ahead—yes! The stew base—*without any seafood*—can be made 2 days ahead and stored in the refrigerator, covered. When ready to serve, bake the fish and bring the stew to a simmer, then add the seafood—shrimp, scallops, clams, and mussels.

This happens fast. When the clams and mussels open—get everyone to the table.

Corn Chowder Delight

Ideal with the fresh summer corn ... or hit the large frozen bag in your grocery story or at Costco. This is for those who love corn—count me in. I always make a big batch and freeze for a I'm not cooking tonight ... I'm tired tonight ... It's cold outside ... Comfort food today please! This was inspired by my Heart Sister Glenda. Hint: prep all veggies before starting.

Serves 10 to 12
ingredients

- 1 stick of butter (equals ½ C)
- 5 T flour
- 1 large onion
- 4-6 celery stalks, cut in slices
- 4 C russet potatoes, peeled and chopped
- 4 C frozen corn. *Do not use canned corn.*
- 2 red bell peppers, chopped
- 1 can Ortega chilis, diced
  If you like a bit more kick, another can
- 4 T sugar
- 4 tsp salt
- 1½ tsp pepper
- 6 C Half and Half. *Don't use milk.*
- 2 avocados. *Cut up for topping at serving*

putting it all together

Melt butter, add flour and whisk—add onion whisk together in large pot. Add and celery and saute under low heat for around 5 minutes.

Bring all ingredients together in big pot. Simmer for 30-40 minutes until potatoes are tender.

Add Half and Half. Only add until soup is hot and thickens—usually less than 15 minutes.

I like to add a fried onion mix as a topping, for added crunch. Melt butter in frying pan, add onions and celery. Sauté until crunch.

Add a salad and favorite biscuit—like Red Lobster's—or bread for dipping. I like a sourdough bread.

Top with avocado small chunks to serve.

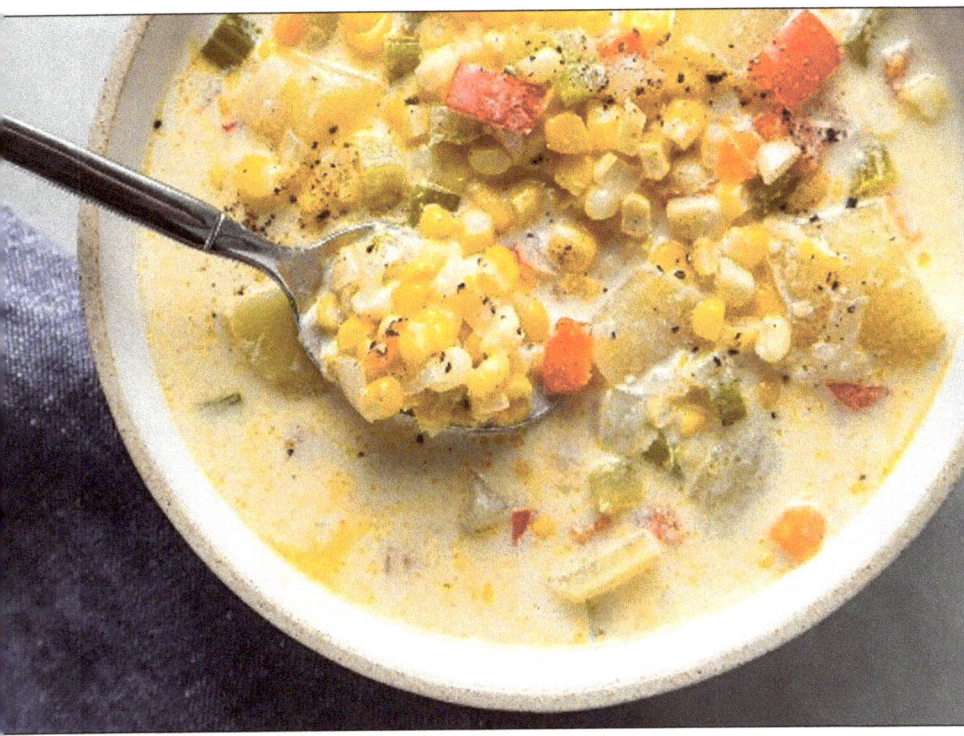

Gazpacho

Gazpacho is a cold soup, loaded with veggies, and summertime favorite. Great drink accompaniments are Sangria and Margaritas. If I'm doing a Mexican spread, Gazpacho is a must-have along with chili relleno casserole, enchiladas, taquitos, and lots of guacamole.

Gazpacho can be served as a main, BUT my preference is as an appetizer. When I do this, I serve it in small glasses—a tad bigger that a double shot glass. Have a basket of tortilla chips close by. It's easy peasy to have a tray of these all ready for guests to pick up and enjoy. Don't be surprised to see seconds grabbed for!

Recommended … do this a day ahead.

Prep time: about 30-40 minutes—chop time!
Servings: 10-12 cups

ingredients

> 7 medium tomatoes (about 3 pounds), peeled and seeded
>
> 2 cucumbers (English best), peeled, halved, seeded, and coarsely chopped—*save some for garnish*
>
> 1 red or green bell pepper, coarsely chopped— *my preferences is for red*
>
> 1 yellow bell pepper, coarsely chopped—*save some for garnish*
>
> 1 small red onion, coarsely chopped
>
> 4 garlic cloves, chopped
>
> ¼ C chopped parsley--save whole leaves for garnish
>
> 6 basil leaves—*add more for garnish*
>
> 1 tsp dried basil
>
> 1 tsp dried oregano
>
> ½ C extra-virgin olive oil
>
> ¼ C red wine vinegar
>
> 1½ T Worcestershire sauce

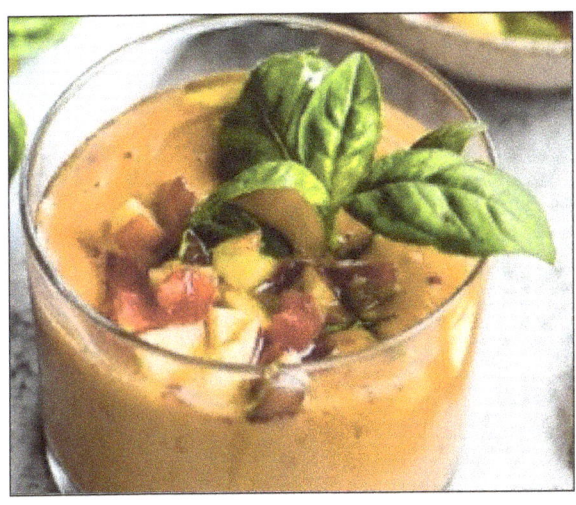

2 T fresh lemon juice

1 T tabasco

One 46-oz jar tomato juice

salt to taste

black pepper, freshly ground, to taste

putting it all together

Chop yellow bell pepper, cucumber and snipped chives or basil for garnish—set aside.

In a large bowl, toss the tomatoes with the cucumbers, red or green bell pepper, onion, garlic, chopped parsley, fresh basil, dried basil, oregano, olive oil, red wine vinegar, Worcestershire sauce, lemon juice, and tabasco.

In a blender, puree the mixture in batches until nearly smooth. Transfer to a large bowl. Stir in the tomato juice and season with salt and pepper. Refrigerate the gazpacho for at least 4 hours or overnight.

Season the soup again if necessary and transfer to bowls or small glasses. Garnish with cucumber, yellow bell pepper, chives and parsley leaves and serve.

The gazpacho can be refrigerated for up to 2 days.

Judith's Chili Relleno Corn Chowder

This is one of the recipes that I included in the first book of the Silver Magnolia series, The Buffet Goes Off the Track *that Izzy serves to her friends as they settled into an afternoon and evening of friendship and puzzles.*

8 Hearty Servings: a meal, add a salad, add some tortilla chips
All cooking is your large stove-top pot.

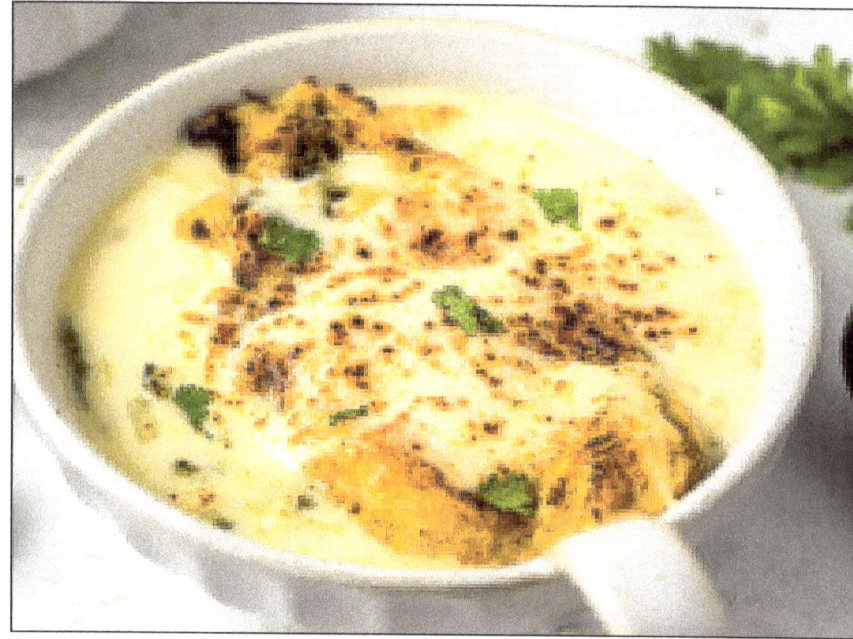

ingredients

½ pound bacon, cut up

2 C yellow or white onions, chopped. *I like the Vidalia.*

8 C chicken broth to pot.
I love Better than Bouillion® chicken flavor.

2 russet potatoes, peeled & chopped

6 ribs of organic celery, chopped

2 4 oz cans Ortega or Hatch diced chilies; *I use Ortega.*

4 T butter

32 oz frozen corn

3 T honey powder

3 C half & half or full creme. *I do both, 1½ C of each*

1 to 1½ C shredded cheddar or Mexican cheeses

4-6 T corn meal.

Salt and pepper to taste.

2 avocados. *Cut for color and taste if you like avocados.*

cilantro

putting it all together

All cooking will be done in a large pot. Cook bacon with onions until the onions start to soften. Add chicken broth, potatoes, celery, chilies, butter, corn, and honey power. Bring to a simmer and allowing the flavors mix.

Blend in the half-in-half and cheese.

Make slurry with corn meal and in one cup of hot water to break down before adding to all for the final blending. This thickens the chowder and enhances the corn flavor. Add salt and pepper to taste.

Optional toppings: avocados and cilantro.

Judith's Easy Peasy French Onion Soup

French Onion Soup is one of those dishes that when I make it, it's as though I forgot how delicious and filling it is ... and why did I wait so long in between soup pots. It's the perfect soup when I feel cold or know the cold is coming in. The aromas in the kitchen are wonderful and the taste sensational.

Serves 4

Full prep plus cooking time is 40 minutes or less.

ingredients

> 3 large onions, cut vertically
>
> 3 T butter
>
> ½ tsp sugar
>
> 1 T flour
>
> salt and pepper, not much
>
> 4 C beef broth, *I use Better than Bouillon® and add to water*
>
> 2 T Worchester sauce
>
> ½ C wine, optional
>
> swiss cheese or gruyere slices
>
> french bread, *I butter and toast just a bit under broiler*
>
> Parmesan cheese, sprinkle this

putting it all together

Heat butter over medium-high heat in large pan. Add onions and sauté for 15 minutes or until tender. Stir frequently. Add sugar, pepper, salt, flour. Reduce heat to medium. Stir in wine if used and cook for 1 minute. Add broth—simmer, covered for 20 minutes.

Broiler. Place buttered bread in a single layer on a baking sheet; broil until toasted. It happens quickly so be vigilant; check every 20 seconds. *I don't turn them, but you can for full toasted effect.*

Use ovenproof bowls on a baking sheet. Ladle soup into each bowl. Place toasted bread on top; add Parmesan cheese then slice of swiss or gruyere on top. Broil 2 minutes or until cheese begins to brown.

Another option is to skip the toasted butter bread and instead, top the soup with fresh baked croutons.

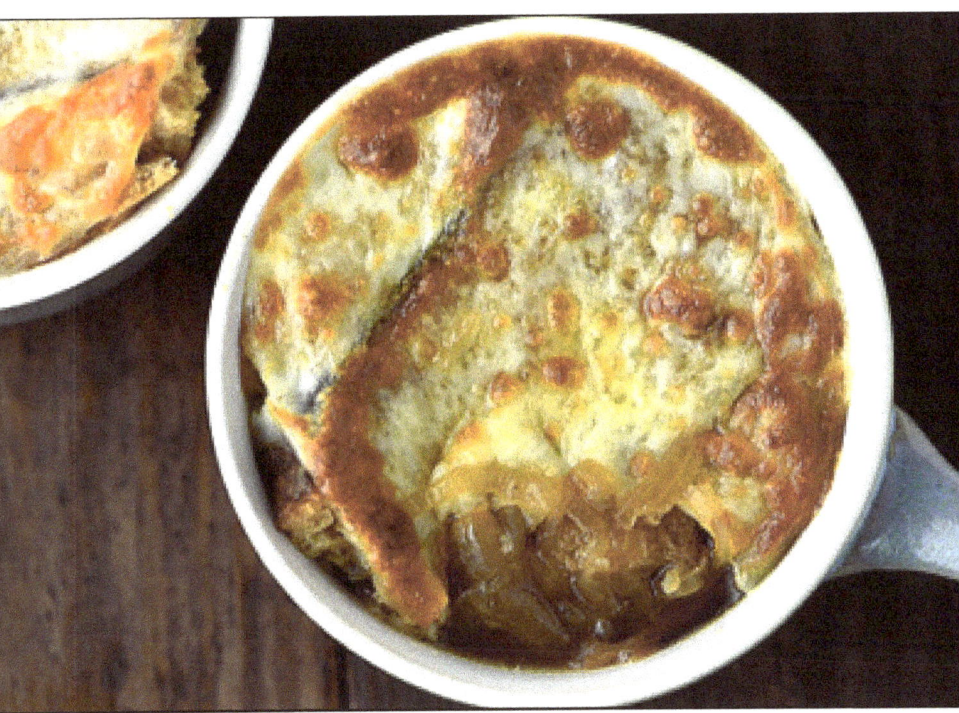

Pumpkin Soup

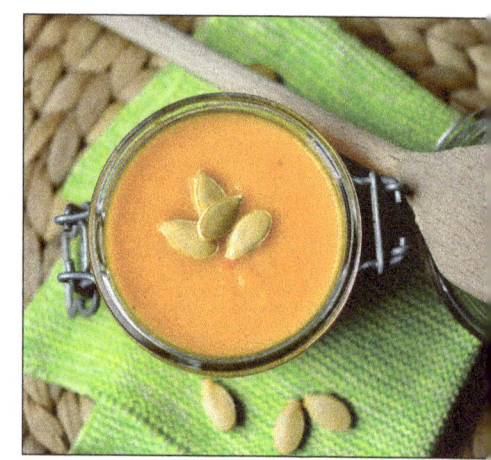

Serves 8 to 10

ingredients

2 T olive or avocado oil, *I usually use avocado oil*

2 onions, diced

2 apples, Granny Smith or Fuji, peeled and diced

2 carrots, diced

½ tsp each of ginger, ground coriander, ground cumin

1 quart chicken broth

1 C coconut milk. (If lactose intolerant—sub in almond milk)

1 (30 oz) can of pumpkin or 2 (15 oz) cans

sour cream or Crème fraîche. (for garnish)

toasted pumpkin seeds (for garnish)

Preheat oven to 350°

putting it all together

Sauté in oil onions, apples, carrots until tender. Add spices. Add broth, coconut milk, and pumpkin. Let simmer 20 to 30 minutes.

Serve with a dollop of sour cream or Crème fraîche.

Sprinkle toasted pumpkin seeds on top. I toast in oven with avocado oil for a few minutes. If you have basil, add a few leaves.

Like crunchies? Add croutons. I like to make crouton baguette slices.

Crouton Baguette Slices, *perfect for dipping in soups*

1 baguette, sliced in ½ inches

Cookie sheet … add olive oil or avocado oil and spread over sheet. Sprinkle slices with powdered garlic or garlic salt. Bake for about 10 minutes.

Red Pepper and Tomato Soup with Croutons

Any time you can get red bell peppers, it's a good time to think of a hearty soup. Add tomatoes, onions, feta cheese (adds to creaminess), seasonings, and a splash of hot sauce—perfect. Bake all the veggies on a cookie sheet, blend and TaDah! Thanks to my friend, author Rox Burkey, for sharing some of the elements to make this delicious, no brainer soup. Add homemade croutons for a perfect, light meal.

This one is an easy peasy. All veggies are baked on a large cookie sheet, then dropped into a whirl in the blender. To add a bit of a kick, include your favorite hot sauce to taste. Ideal to have in your freezer for a quick defrost and reheat.

Veggie cooking: 40-45 minutes in 400° oven. Cookie sheet bake, then blender.

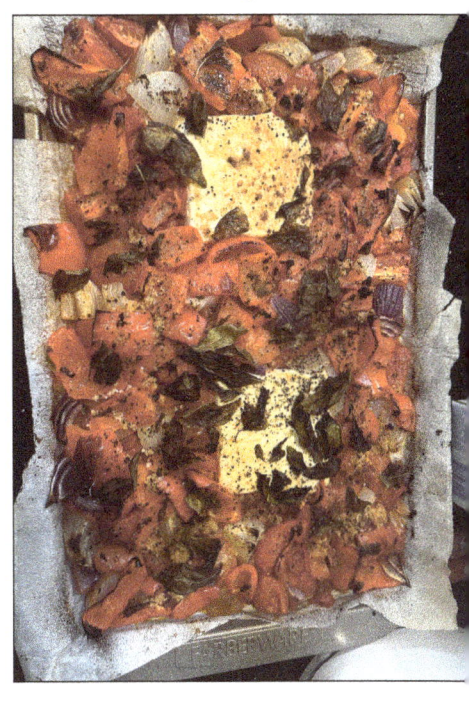

ingredients

- 6 red bell peppers
- 8 Roma tomatoes
- 2 red onions
- 2 sweet onions
- 4 cloves garlic
- 1 C basil leaves
- 2 8 oz feta cheese blocks
- 6 C broth. *I use Better than Bouillon® vegetable flavor.*

olive oil, garlic salt, cumin, hot sauce— *I always have Cholula in my pantry.*

continued

putting it all together

Prep your cookie sheets … have two of them with parchment paper. Seed peppers and cut in large pieces; same with onions and tomatoes. Add garlic. Spread across cookie sheets, add feta cheese into center and generous amounts of basil. Add generous drizzles of olive oil over your mixture—salt, pepper, cumin to taste.

To the oven for 40-45 minutes. When done, add veggies and the broth to your blender and run until smooth—it will be THICK. Don't forget to add the drippings from the cookie sheet. If you want a little "kick," add hot sauce to taste when blending.

Meanwhile … make your croutons

　　1 baguette

　　olive oil or avocado oil

　　garlic salt

Cut baguette into pieces. I slice the entire baguette into ½ inch thick slices, than divide again into six pieces … olive or avocado oil on cookie sheet; add garlic salt to taste. *I'm generous with both.*

Sometimes I'll add in grated Parmesan cheese. Bake in 350° until desired firmness—no more than 10 minutes.

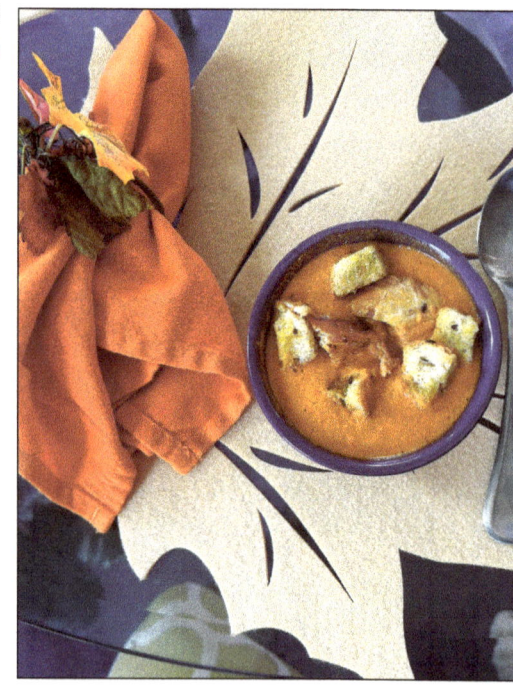

Rustic Italian Tortellini Soup

Think HEARTY when making this. Perfect for cool weather eating as a main course. If you do, add a salad and light dessert. When I first made it, I was the "appetizer course" for one of my foodie groups. A huge hit where all said, "Another helping please … and this could be the main course." Definitely.

Prep: 20 min. Cook: 20 min …

6 servings; 2 quarts
ingredients

¾ pound Italian turkey sausage links, *REMOVE casings*

1 medium onion, chopped

6 garlic cloves, minced

2 cans (14½ ounces each) chicken broth OR create from Better than Bouillon® chicken flavor—*usually my choice*

1¾ C water

1 can (14½ ounces) diced tomatoes, undrained

1 package (9 ounces) refrigerated cheese tortellini

1 package (6 ounces) fresh baby spinach, coarsely chopped

2¼ tsp minced fresh basil or ¾ tsp dried basil

1 red bell pepepr

¼ tsp pepper

Dash crushed red pepper flakes

Shredded Parmesan cheese (optional)

putting it all together

Crumble sausage into a Dutch oven; add onion. Most sausage has fat in it. If you need moisture, add 1 T oil or butter. Cook and stir over medium heat until meat is no longer pink. Add garlic; cook 1 minute longer.

continued

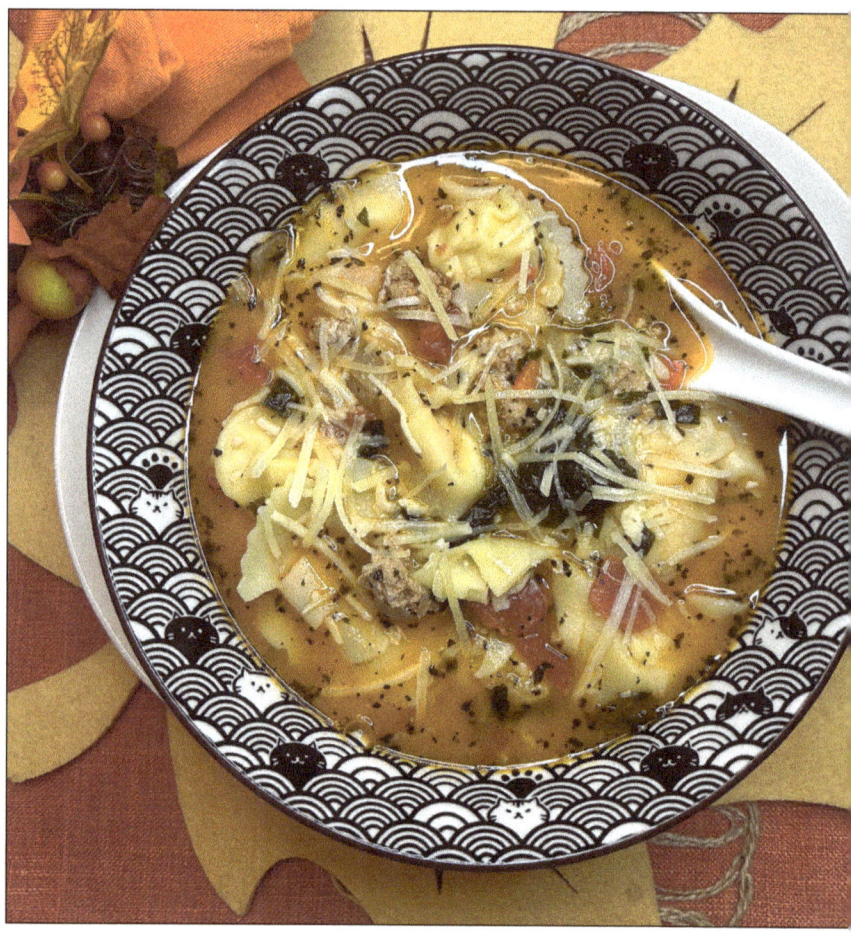

Stir in broth, water, and tomatoes. Bring to a boil. Add tortellini; return to a boil. Cook for 5-8 minutes or until almost tender, stirring occasionally.

Reduce heat; add the spinach, basil, bell pepper, and pepper flakes. Cook 2-3 minutes longer or until spinach is wilted and tortellini are tender. Serve immediately with Parmesan cheese.

Freeze option: Place individual portions of cooled soup in freezer containers and freeze. To use, partially thaw in refrigerator overnight. Heat through in a saucepan, stirring occasionally and adding a little broth if necessary.

Avocado Corn Salad
Plain, Chicken, or Shrimp

Perfect for Spring through Fall times. As a side ... or consider adding diced chicken or cold cooked shrimp and make it a main course meal. If you love corn, cilantro, and avocado, this salad is for you.

Serves 4

ingredients

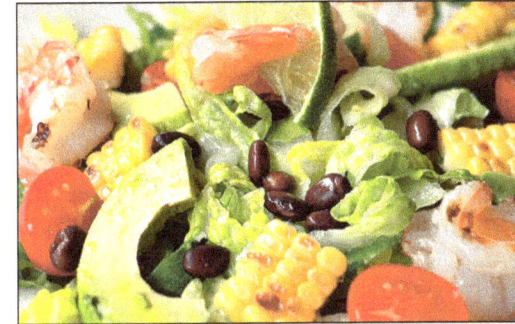

6 ears of corn, fresh or frozen *(never canned)*

1 C diced chicken or 1 cup cold shrimp *(both optional)*

⅓ to ½ red onion, chopped

green onions, chopped, plus some to sprinkle on top

salt and chile powder ... *as much as you want*

cilantro, ¼ head, loosely torn, plus more as a topping

avocado

1 T lime juice

dash of olive oil

putting it all together

Cook corn on the cob on the grill or boil in a pot of water. This can be done ahead of time and kept in the refrigerator, in an air-tight container. OR if using frozen, thaw, then cook for a few minutes in boiling water. Drain.

In a large bowl, mix corn, chicken or shrimp (if using), red and green onions. Add salt and chili powder. Add cilantro. *Some can't tolerate cilantro. I love it. Always have it in a separate bowl guests can add to their salad.*

In small bowl, add diced avocado, lime juice, and olive oil. Gently mix until evenly incorporated.)

Add avocado mixture to corn and mix. Sprinkle green onions and cilantro on top to finish. Serve right away.

Irresistible Grape Salad

My Heart Sisters Ellen and Glenda refer to this as "crack grapes"—oh my! Eat one … and who knows how many will follow.

ingredients
4 pounds clean seedless grapes, patted dry. Leave whole. *Freshest grapes best. Mix green and red.*

combine
8 oz cream cheese, softened

8 oz sour cream

½ C sugar or Splenda

1 tsp vanilla

2 drops orange oil (optional, at Sprouts)

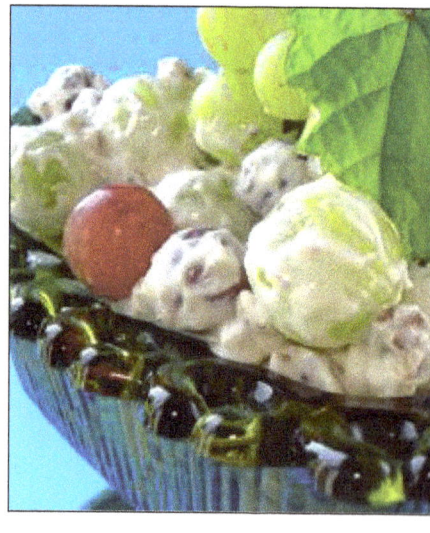

putting it all together
Mix until smooth. Fold in grapes and stir gently. Make sure to cover all the grapes with the mixture.

Pour into 9" x 13" dish or pan.

topping
1 C brown sugar

1 C pecans, finely chopped

In small bowl, mix brown sugar and pecans.

Cover grapes with pecan topping.

Cover dish and chill at least 2 hours. *Gets better over time.*

Judith's 24-Hour Salad

Prep: 30 minutes max
24 hours in the refrigerator

ingredients

2 bell peppers—your choice: green, red, yellow, orange

1 C corn

1 C celery, diced

1 red onion, diced

1 C peas—frozen

2 heads iceberg lettuce, chopped

2 C mayonnaise

½ C Parmesan, grated

salt and pepper to taste

1 pound bacon, cooked and diced

1 C cheddar cheese, grated, if you like on top

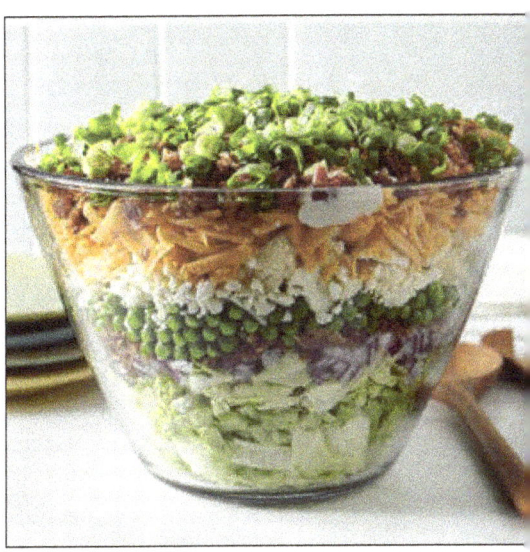

putting it all together

Layer first 6 ingredients listed above with lettuce on bottom. In small bowl, mix mayo, Parmesan, salt and pepper; add bacon and cheddar cheese. Cover bowls and refrigerate.

Next day … I dump the two bowls into a big bowl and mix it all up with my hands. *It's great as leftover.*

Judith's Apple or Pear Pecan Salad with Honey Mustard Dressing

This is a HUGE hit salad! Super fast to put together—less than 10 minutes. Dressing takes about 5 minutes. A perfect beginning for a fall gathering and festive with its colors for the Holidays. Many times, my guests ask for more.

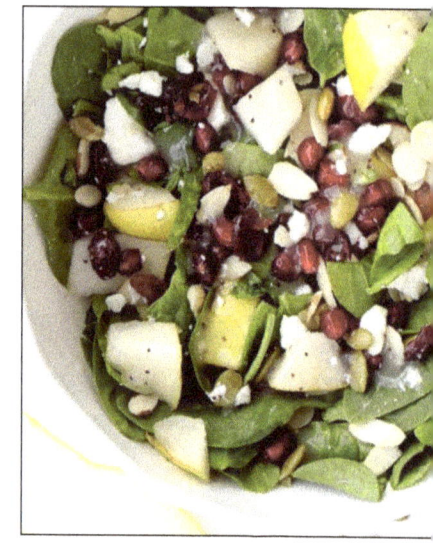

Serves 8
ingredients

2 pears, Red D 'Anjou, sliced

2 apples, Fuji or Honey Crisp, sliced

1 red leaf lettuce head, torn

12 oz baby spinach

1 C pomegranate seeds

½ C dried cranberries

¾ C pumpkin seeds, roasted

optional

½ C slivered almonds, roasted

6 oz Feta or Gorgonzola cheese. *I prefer a Hungarian or French Feta I find in Middle Eastern grocery stores … and love, love Gorgonzola. Pick one!*

putting it all together

Place all of the ingredients in a large salad bowl. Drizzle with the desired amount of honey mustard dressing and gently toss.

Serve immediately!

Honey Mustard Dressing

ingredients

¼ C Dijon mustard

3 T honey *or more to taste*

3 T apple cider vinegar *or more to taste*

1 T fresh lemon juice (optional)

¼ to ½ tsp fine sea salt

¼ tsp fresh ground black pepper

¼ C extra virgin olive oil

putting it all together

Combine the mustard, honey, apple cider vinegar, lemon juice, ¼ teaspoon salt, and the black pepper and whisk until well blended and creamy.

Whisk in the oil, and then taste the dressing. I keep in a mason jar with lid and shake well.

If you want more tartness, adjust with additional salt, vinegar, or honey. If you want even more tart, add another tsp of vinegar. If you want less tartness, reduce vinegar.

Judith's Summer Beet Salad

My version—I discovered this at CheeseCake Factory and then did my own tweaking. One of my dinner deck guests took one bite, and then pulled the entire platter to him. "I'll have this for my dinner!" Maybe I should call it Dan's Beet Salad?

Serves 4
Prep: less than 10 minutes (love this)
ingredients

pickled beets, already sliced. *I use ½ a jar*

1 orange

2 avocado, sliced

yogurt with honey. *I got at Kroger's King Sooper. If you can't find, get vanilla yogurt, add two tablespoons of honey.*

Crispy onions ... add just before serving—great crunch. *I use French's Fried Onions.*

putting it all together

Spread a generous portion of yogurt on bottom of serving platter. Add a generous layer of beets on top of yogurt. Top with cut up orange; then add sliced avocado. Just before serving, sprinkle crispy onions on top.

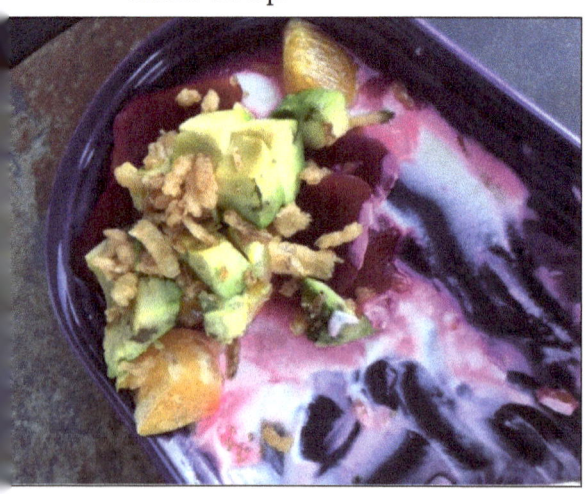

That's it ... easy, peasy and delicious! I put together all but the crispy onions about 30 minutes before serving and chill in refrigerator, ready for table.

Lobster Salad

I love lobster. Any lobster. My personal record was devouring five small Maine lobsters that were barbequed on a sand dune in Maine. Baked, boiled, cold—it doesn't matter. When I do lobster tails, I make an extra, or two, for later. The "later" will become a delectable salad—or lobster rolls with hot dog buns! For the salad, I love a warm piece of Sourdough bread. Add your favorite white wine … or for me, a tall, iced tea. When I first made this, John cleaned his plate—"Delicious," was all that came out of his mouth.

Lobster cooking

If you are boiling your whole lobsters or the tails, fill your pot with hot water and add herbs and spices—several sprigs of parsley, peppercorns, one tsp of paprika, maybe a bay leaf or two, 3 lemons squeezed for the juice, 2 cloves of garlic, 1 tsp red pepper flakes. You will cook for around 8-9 minutes, depending on the size. Pull out, cool to room temperature and crack to get the meat out. You will need strong scissors to break through the shell. Cut into bite size pieces.

If baking your lobster, you are going to split the lobster on the outer curved side and pop out the meat. At this point, I have melted butter with garlic as a baster. Cook for about 8-9 minutes. Cool to room temperature and cut into bite size pieces.

Serves 4 … plus warm Sourdough Garlic bread

continued

For Salad ... Lunch or Dinner

ingredients

1 C mayonnaise

1 tsp garlic powder

2 tsp Dijon mustard

2 tsp sweet chili sauce

½ fresh squeeze lemon juice

½ C celery, diced

½ C champagne vinegar

2 tsp minced fresh tarragon, *dried is also OK*

2 tsp minced fresh chives, plus more for serving

Salt and Pepper to taste

3 lobster tails

putting it all together

Mix all together. Add lobster. This is a moist salad … not dry.

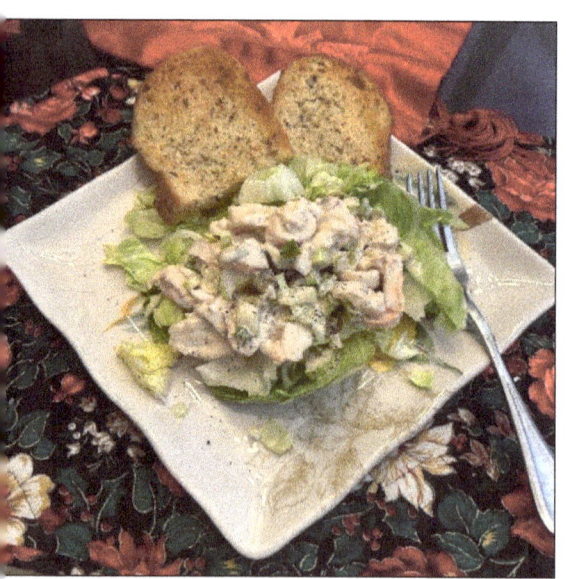

Lemon – sliced at serving, optional … Definitely warm Sourdough garlic bread.

Butter lettuce leaves, for serving into—I also use ½ of iceberg, and chop into salad. You may want to have sliced lemon to squeeze over finished serving—eater's choice.

Mardi Gras Salad

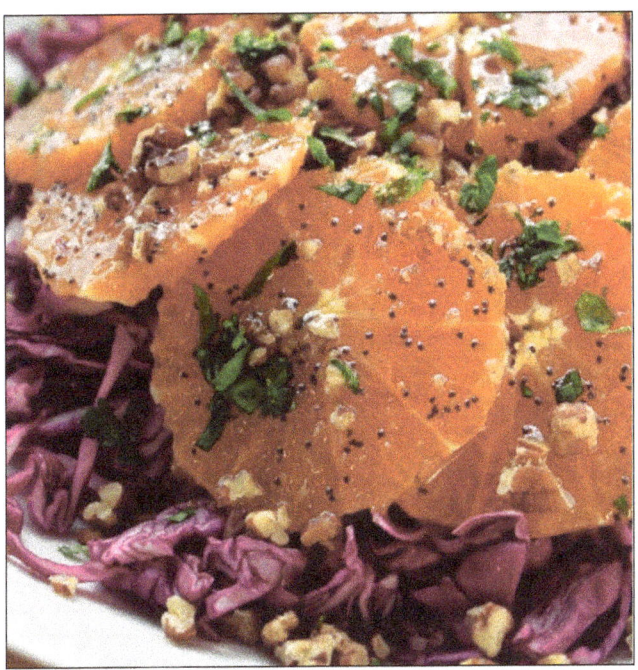

One of my foodie groups declared Mardi Gras theme for the evening cooking soiree. Whatever dish we were bringing—main, appetizer, sides, or dessert—it had to be a connected to Mardi Gras. I was the chef for the sides and had an idea for a simple, but tasty salad. The orange, red cabbage, and pecan combination was perfect for spring weather.

serves 6 – 8
ingredients

- 3 navel oranges, peeled and sliced
- 4 C red cabbage, thinly sliced
- ¼ C pecans or pistachios, chopped snd toasted
- 2 T parsley, chopped
- ½ C poppy seed dressing

continued

poppy seed dressing ingredients

    1 C olive oil

    ½ C red wine vinegar

    ¼ C sweet white wine

    2 T soy sauce

    1 T Dijon mustard

    2 T poppy seeds

putting it all together

Start with the dressing. Whisk the olive oil, red wine vinegar, white wine, and soy sauce together. Add the mustard and blend. Mix in the poppy seeds and put aside.

Then the salad. Peel the oranges. Do not separate the sections—you will cross cut the orange for multiple slices. Trim any excess white membrane, known as the pith, from the fruit. You just want the juicy orange slice.

In a bowl, add the thinly sliced red cabbage, pecans or pistachios, parsley, and the orange slices. Add your dressing and serve.

Pears and Pomegranates Red Leaf Lettuce Salad

This was a big hit when I first presented it during the Holidays with friends. A salad where my friends asked for another serving. It's a visual delight.

Serves 8

salad ingredients

- 1 medium head red leaf lettuce, torn
- 1 medium butter lettuce, torn
- 1-2 Bosc pears, thinly slice
- ¾ C goat cheese, crumbled
- ⅓ C pomegranate seeds
- ½ C pecans, toasted

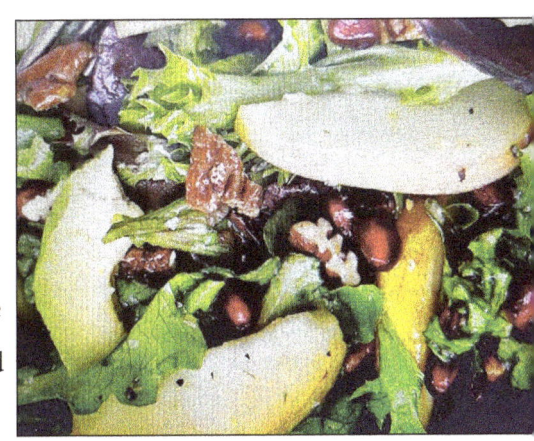

vinaigrette ingredients

- 3 T extra-virgin olive oil
- 3 T balsamic vinegar
- 2 T honey
- 1 clove minced garlic
- ½ tsp kosher salt
- freshly ground black pepper to taste

putting it all together

Whisk together the olive oil, balsamic vinegar, honey, garlic, salt and pepper in a small bowl. Gently toss with torn lettuces.

Top with pear slices, goat cheese, pomegranate seeds, and pecans.

Red and Green Christmas Salad

I made this salad for the first time last year. It was a big hit with my family and friends. The pomegranate red and kiwi green colors have a festive flair, and pomegranates are excellent this time of year. To save time on Christmas Day, I opened a fresh pomegranate the day before following the directions shared here and stored the seeds in a covered container in the refrigerator overnight.

Serves 4

for the dressing

4 T balsamic vinegar

4 T olive oil

Place balsamic vinegar in a small bowl and slowly whisk in the olive oil. Continue to whisk until emulsified. Cover and refrigerate until ready to serve.

for the salad

1 head red leaf and/or butter lettuce, washed, dried, and torn into bite-size pieces

4 kiwis, peeled and each cut into 6 wedges

½ C pomegranate seeds

2 T pine nuts, toasted

4 T Gorgonzola cheese, crumbled.

putting it all together

Cover 4 salad plates with lettuce. In the middle of the salad plates, arrange kiwi wedges in a circular pattern. Sprinkle each salad with pomegranate seeds, pine nuts, and Gorgonzola cheese. Drizzle dressing over salad. Do not toss. Serve immediately.

tips for buying

Do not buy any fruit that has cracks on its skin. It's overripe. Pomegranates are "heavy" and you want the fruit firm. Buy ahead. Pomegranates become juicier and have more flavor over time.

to open a pomegranate

Cut off the crown. Divide the pomegranate into quarters. Pull the four sections apart. Remove all the white pith and discard. Now, flip the pomegranate inside out and pop the seeds out by pushing skin.

If you still have some of the white pith, place the quartered sections into a bowl of cold water. The seeds will sink to the bottom.

Watermelon Salad with Feta and Cucumber-Mint

Perfect for the summertime. Summertime is deck and garden time for me. I promise … it's refreshing and will disappear fast.

Prep Time less than 15 minutes
Serves 4, so double, etc., for more
ingredients

> 3 C watermelon cubed or balled
>
> 1 ½ C sliced cucumber seeds removed
>
> 2 tablespoons mint, thinly sliced or small mint leaves
>
> ½ C feta cheese crumbled. *I use French Feta from a local Middle Eastern grocery*
>
> 3 T olive oil
>
> 1 T lime juice
>
> salt and pepper to taste

dressing
In a small bowl, whisk together the olive oil, lime juice, salt and pepper.

putting it all together
Place the watermelon, cucumber, and mint in a large bowl.

Drizzle the dressing over the melon mixture and toss to coat.

Add the feta and serve.

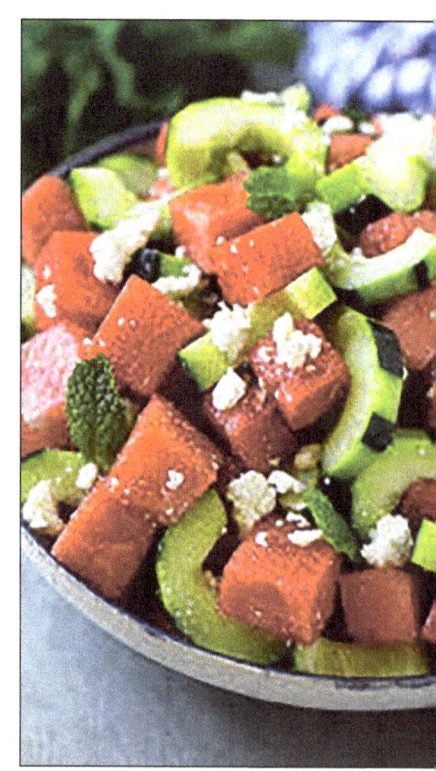

Asiago Bacon Capers and Garlic Roasted Asparagus

Cooking time: 15 minutes

ingredients

- 1–2 pounds asparagus, trim ends
- 2–3 T olive oil
- capers, a few tablespoons
- 4 garlic cloves, minced
- 1 C grated Asiago cheese
- 4 bacon slices, cooked, drained of fat, chopped
- salt and pepper, if desired

Preheat oven to 425°

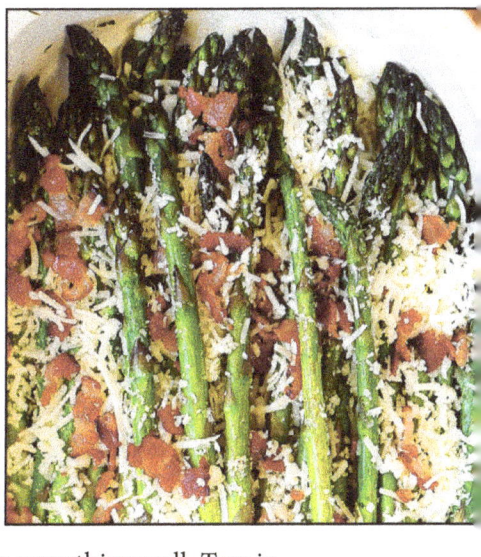

putting it all together

Place asparagus in casserole dish or baking sheet. Drizzle with olive oil and season with salt and pepper. Mix everything well. Toss in minced garlic.

Roast for 10 minutes, uncovered. REMOVE from oven.

Sprinkle half of grated Asiago cheese over asparagus. Add chopped, cooked bacon. Top with capers and the remaining grated Asiago cheese.

Roast for 5 more minutes, uncovered.

Buttery Garlic Mushrooms

If you are a fan of mushrooms, kissed with butter and garlic ... this will become a favorite with family and friends. When I bring it to my Foodie group, I always make extra for them to take home. Great with an omelet the next day, on hamburgers, or in rice.

Whole onions are sliced, butter added to caramelize with garlic, cremini, baby portobello, and shiitake mushrooms are sauteed with fresh garlic, caramelized onions, salt, and pepper. This easy side dish comes together in less than 20 minutes, including your prep time. Enjoy!

Serves 8

ingredients

- 10-12 oz mushrooms of each: sliced cremini, shiitake, and baby portobello
- 2 vidalia onions. *I prefer sweet*
- 2 T olive oil
- 2 T butter
- 8 cloves garlic, minced
- 1 tsp salt
- ½ tsp black pepper
- Parsley, for garnish

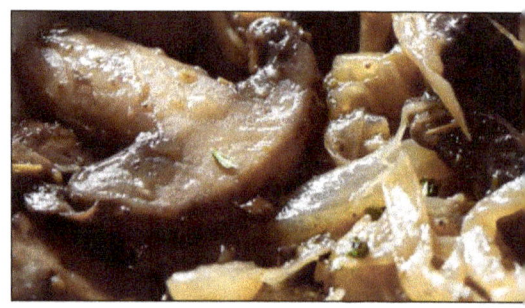

putting it all together

In pan, add olive oil and butter, and sliced onions. Cook to simmer for caramelizing. Set aside.

Gently clean mushrooms and cut stems. Dry. In another pan, add olive oil and butter and garlic. Simmer until cooked. Add onions and seasonings. Serve immediately.

Fingerlings

I first did this for a Holiday dinner with my Foodie Friends. It was a hit, along with the Buttery Garlic Mushrooms. Fingerlings are eye appealing with the white and red potatoes usually in the mix from your grocery store. Their texture is almost creamy in your mouth. The great thing about fingerlings is that you can do prep work the day before—cut and store in a bag with water.

Leftovers? Think breakfast the next day with eggs on top.

Cooking time: 20 minutes
Serves 8
ingredients

> 2 pounds total in weight fingerlings, cut in half lengthwise … *even the small ones*
>
> 2 lemons, zest. *You will zest into your mixture to coat*
>
> 3 cloves of garlic, minced
>
> ½ – ¾ C Parmesan cheese
>
> 3 T butter
>
> 3 T olive oil
>
> 1 tsp salt
>
> 1 tsp black pepper
>
> 3-4 T parsley, as garnish

Preheat oven to 425°

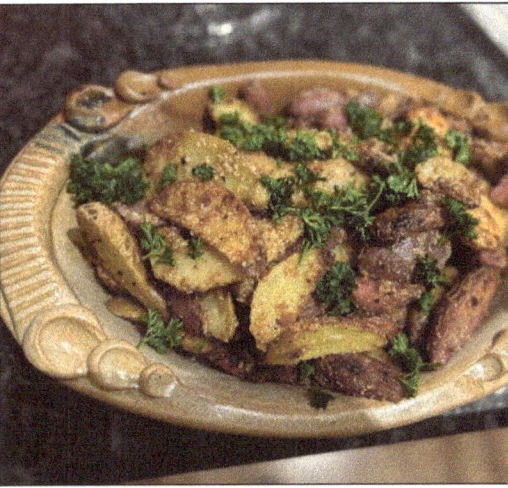

putting it all together
When ready to do your baking, Mix all ingredients together in a large bowl. Add the fingerlings. Lay out on a cookie sheet. Drizzle with a little more olive oil if needed and into the oven until cooked.

Mardi Gras Maque Choux

Get ready to enjoy a tasty side dish. Works in all seasons. The first time I prepared this was at my foodie group's Mardi Gras themed dinner. I was responsible for all the sides.

Prep: 35 min. | Cook: 30 mins
Serves 6

ingredients

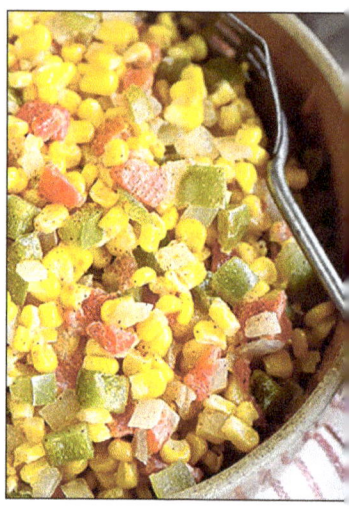

- 6 ears of fresh corn, husked and cleaned – or frozen
- 2 T vegetable oil
- 1 large onion, thinly sliced
- 1 C green or red bell pepper, chopped
- 1 large fresh tomato, chopped
- ¼ C milk
- salt to taste
- cayenne pepper
- ¼ C chopped green onions
- 8 strips crisply cooked bacon, crumbled

putting it all together

Cut corn off the cobs or thaw frozen corn; place in a medium bowl. **Cutting across kernels releases milk** from the corn.
Add the ¼ cup milk to bowl. Set aside.

Heat the oil in a large skillet over medium-high heat. Add onion and green pepper. Cook until onion is transparent, about 5 to 8 minutes. Combine corn, tomatoes, and milk with the onion mixture. Reduce heat to medium low, and cook 20 minutes longer, stirring frequently to prevent sticking. Do not boil.

Season with salt and cayenne pepper. Lower heat, cover skillet, and cook 5 to 10 minutes longer. Stir in green onions and bacon. Remove from heat and serve.

Orzo and Wild Rice

I first had this when my friend Steve was the "side dish" person for my foodie group. I loved it, and then started to tinker a bit, adding a few more ingredients. It's a perfect side dish for a main course.

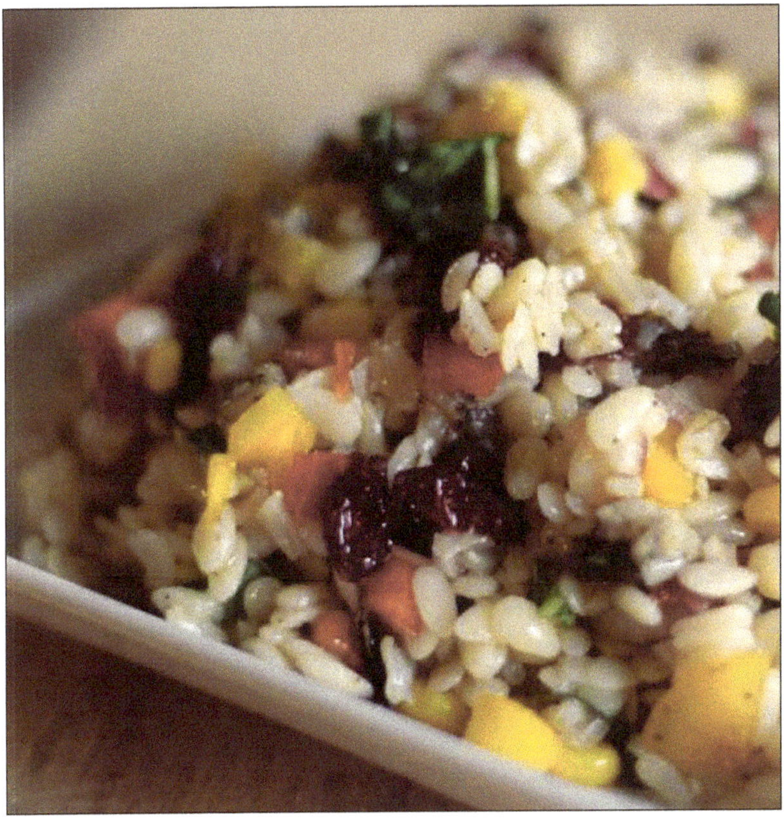

ingredients

- 5 C cooked orzo
- 3 C cooked wild rice
- ½ C chopped parsley
- ½ small red onion, diced
- 6 T currants
- 1 C corn, *I use frozen ... fresh is welcomed*

continued

1 each red of orange and yellow peppers, diced small

1 tsp dill, *fresh is always good*

½ C roasted pecans

dressing ingredients

1 C of good olive oil

¼ C white balsamic vinegar

3 T honey

½ T Dijon mustard

1 tsp minced garlic

1 tsp fresh basil or 1 T fresh basil, minced

1 tsp Kosher salt

1 tsp black pepper

putting it all together

Place all the ingredients in a mixing bowl, except the olive oil. Stir until blended and then while whisking the dressing, slowly pour the olive oil in a steady stream. Refrigerate.

Cook the orzo and wild rice according to package directions, shock in cold water and then refrigerate.

Put all ingredients into a large mixing bowl and toss with the dressing.

Refrigerate for at least an hour or two so the dressing can soak into the ingredients.

Pearl Onion and Cheese au Gratin

This is unexpected side dish that is bursting with wonderful flavors! Gussy-up your Holiday tables. Also works well with fall and winter comfort meals.

ingredients

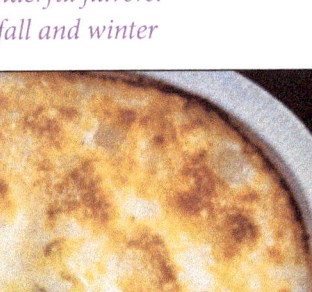

2 10-ounce packages frozen pearl onions

4 T butter

2 T all-purpose flour

1½ C half-and-half

½ tsp salt

½ tsp freshly ground black pepper

¼ tsp ground mustard

Dash of ground nutmeg

2 C (9 oz.) shredded Cheddar cheese, yellow or white

1¼ C fresh breadcrumbs or panko

Preheat oven to 350°

putting it all together

Thaw frozen onions and heat in the microwave or simmer on the stovetop until tender, 3 or 4 minutes. Drain well. Set aside

Melt 2 tablespoons butter in a heavy saucepan over low heat; add flour, stir until smooth and cook for one minute. Over medium heat, gradually add half-and-half, stirring constantly until thickened. Add salt, pepper, mustard, and nutmeg. Add 1½ cups shredded cheese; stir until cheese melts. Gently stir in drained onions. Pour onion mixture into a lightly greased 1-quart baking dish. Sprinkle with the remaining ½ cup of shredded cheese.

Toss breadcrumbs with melted butter until crumbs are well coated. Sprinkle evenly over cheese. Bake, uncovered, for 25 to 30 minutes, or until thoroughly heated and top is golden.

Slow-Cooker Creamed Corn

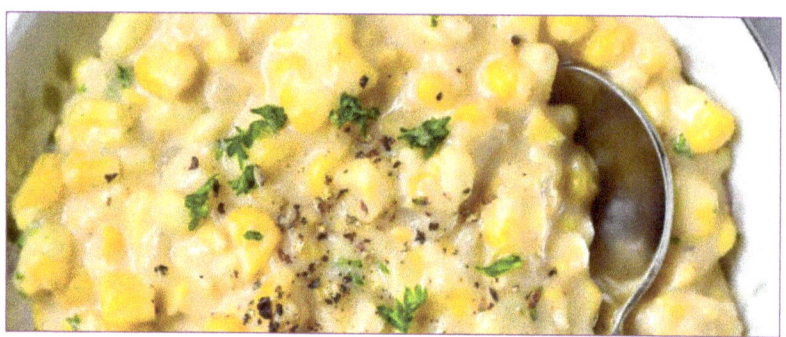

Creamy Corn is a huge pot of taste bud comfort and easy peasy. Expect seconds from your crowd when you serve. Perfect for large groups, holidays. I like to leave it in the crock pot so it stays warm until the last spoonful is taken. Always a hit—yummers!

Serves 8 - 12

ingredients

    32 – 48 ounces frozen white and yellow corn (not canned or fresh)

    8 – 12 ounces cream cheese cut into 1-inch cubes

    ½ – 1 C heavy cream

    ½ – 1 C butter

    2 – 3 T sugar

    ½ – 1 tsp black pepper

    ¼ – ½ tsp salt

    ½ C Parmesan cheese

    Garnish with chives and/or cut green onions

putting it all together

Combine all ingredients in the crock-pot and cook on low for 4 hours. Stir to combine and make sure the cream cheese has completely melted into the sauce.

Judith's Mushroom Quiche

When I host a brunch, there is always be quiche. Typically, I make four at a time. Two for the event and the other two to freeze. Fillings vary. Quiches with cheddar are always a hit. I usually add a Quiche Lorraine —fill with bacon, Gruyère cheese or Swiss cheese, and shallots.

First baking: 8 + 4-5 minutes
Second baking: 30-35 minutes
Serves 6-8 depending on serving size
ingredients

- Pillsbury pie crust, roll out and put in pie pan or use a Deep-Dish Frozen shell
- 6–8 pieces bacon cooked, crumbled
- ¼ C butter
- 1 onion, finely chopped
- 6-8 mushrooms, sliced
- 3 eggs, one will be used to brush the pie crust before baking
- 1–1¼ C sour cream, heaping
- ¼ C cream cheese
- ¼ tsp salt
- ⅛ tsp pepper
- 2 C cheddar cheese, grated. *Try Mexican blend*
- Green onions, chopped

Preheat the oven to 450°. You will decrease to 325° after the empty pie shell is baked.

continued

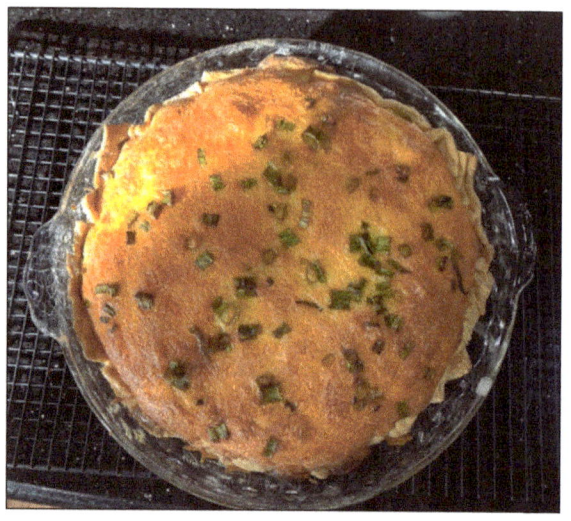

putting it all together

Prick bottom of pie shell and weight the bottom with dried beans or pie weights, Bake for 8 minutes. Remove the dried beans or weights. Cool slightly and brush with beaten egg. Bake another 4-5 minutes. You can add any left over egg to the other two eggs in filling.

Fry bacon, drain and crumble. Discard bacon fat from pan. Sauté onion in ¼ C butter until almost caramelized. Add mushrooms, continue sautéing until softened.

Whisk eggs and add in sour cream, cream cheese, salt and pepper.

Build Quiche in layers: Mushroom/onion mixture in bottom of shell, spread bacon over mushroom/onion mixture; spread generous half of cheddar cheese; pour egg mixture over. Spread remaining cheddar cheese and sprinkle the green onion over top.

Bake at 325° for approximately 35 minutes. If the top of your pie shell is browning too quickly, add a strip of aluminum foil to the edge.

It's done when an inserted knife comes out clean. Wait at least 10 minutes before serving.

Quiche Lorraine

Another favorite on quiche making day—Quiche Lorraine. I make two of these—one for immediate eating, the other for freezing.

First baking: 8 + 4-5 minutes
Second baking: 30-35 minutes
Serves 6-8 depending on serving size
ingredients

    1 9-inch pie pastry.
I prefer deep dish if you get frozen from grocery store

    6 – 8 slices bacon

    1 medium onion, diced

    3 shallots, diced

    2 C shredded Gruyère cheese or Swiss cheese

    2 T all-purpose flour

    3 large eggs, beaten

    1 ½ cups milk or half and half.
I use what I have in the refrigerator

    ½ tsp salt and pepper

    3 T green onions, diced

Preheat the oven to 450°. You will decrease to 325° after the empty pie shell is baked.

putting it all together
Place pie pastry into a 9-inch pie pan; line with a double layer of aluminum foil and a layer of dried beans. If you have pie weights, use those. *I've always done the dried beans.*

Bake pie shell in the preheated oven until golden on the edges, about 8 minutes. Carefully remove the foil and weights; continue baking until crust is set and dry, about 4 minutes more. Remove from the oven and reduce the temperature to 325°. Remove dried beans or weights.

continued

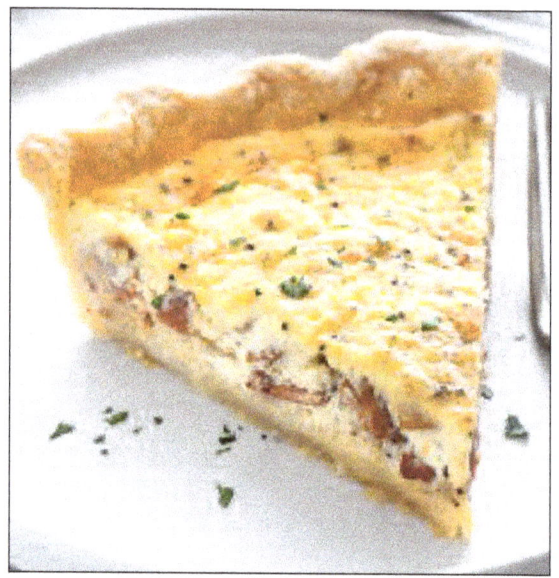

While the crust is baking, cook bacon in a large skillet over medium-high heat until crisp, about 10 minutes. Transfer to a paper towel-lined plate and crumble when cool enough to handle. Drain all but 2 T drippings from the skillet.

Add onion and shallots to drippings in the skillet; cook and stir over medium heat until tender, about 5 minutes. Remove and set aside.

Toss Gruyère or Swiss cheese and flour together in a small bowl.

Whisk milk, eggs, salt and pepper together in a larger bowl, then add in bacon and onion mixture. Mix in cheese mixture until well combined.

Pour into pie crust. Top with a few chopped green onion for a little color.

Bake in the preheated oven until a knife inserted into the center comes out clean, approximately 35 minutes.

If you see your quiche edges over-browning, cover the edge of crust with foil while baking to prevent burning or over-browning.

Let stand for 10 minutes before serving.

Creamy Corn Pasta with Basil and Parmesan

Three steps ... that's all you need to put together a mixed comfort food with fresh summer corn ... or pull from your freezer. Think of it as a side or a full meal. I love corn ... and pasta is one of the ingredients that slides down my throat easily. Basil is one of my favorite herbs, so bring them all together. This is a perfect casual dinner for a movie night. Great at the height of summer corn. And don't forget the kiss of lemon juice.

ingredients

12 oz dry farfalle or orecchiette. *Have some fun with your pasta ... but, this also works with a linguine.*

2 C pasta cooking water—*you will create a sauce with this.*

1 T olive oil, plus extra for drizzling when you serve

1 bunch green scallions, trimmed and thinly sliced— use the cut whites for other dishes.

3 large ears of shucked corn, creates about 2½ C kernels

1 avocado, diced or sliced

½ tsp garlic salt

½ tsp ground black pepper, more for serving

4 T unsalted butter

¾ to 1 C grated Parmesan cheese

½ cup torn basil - more for garnish

¼ tsp red pepper flakes. *If you want more of a kick, add to taste.*

Sea salt to taste

½ lemon, squeezed

continued

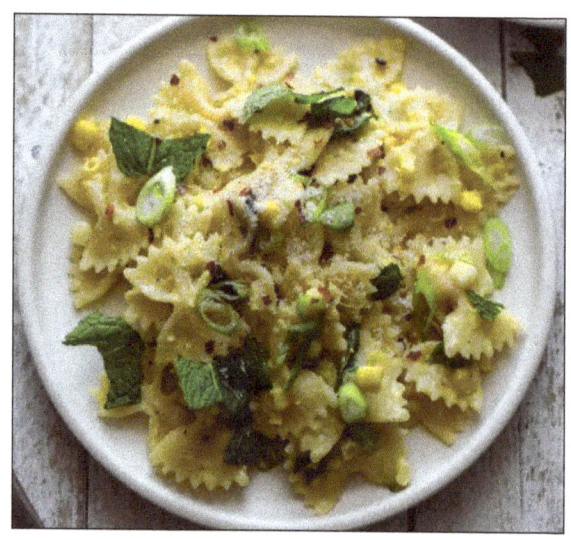

putting it all together

Bring a large pot of water to a boil. Season with a big pinch of salt then add pasta and cook until al dente. Drain all pasta water. Save 2 cups and set aside.

While the pasta is cooking, melt butter in a large skillet. Turn heat down to medium then add sweet corn and garlic, season with more salt and pepper, and then saute until sweet corn is slightly tender—no more than 3 minutes.

Add basil and a small squeeze of lemon juice ... you can always add more later. Stir to combine. If pasta is not done cooking at this point, turn heat down to low under corn.

Once pasta is al dente, transfer pasta into the corn skillet mix and toss to combine. Add Parmesan cheese and 1 C reserved pasta cooking water. Simmer while stirring until a light and creamy sauce has been formed. Add more pasta cooking water if needed to create a light sauce. As it cools, it thickens.

Taste for more salt, pepper, and/or fresh lemon juice if needed. Garnish with a few small basil leaves. I like to add avocado to it as well.

Enjoy ...

Easy Peasy Recipes That Are Quick and Delicious 65

Judith's Baked Spaghetti

An ultimate comfort meal. Typically, after I and have a serving, the left overs are transitioned into what I call "bricks"—I cut small plate servings in pieces that are wrapped for freezing and a thaw and reheat for a quick meal later. With leftovers, I divide into what I call "bricks" and freeze for future meals.

Cook Time: 60 minutes
Serves 8 to 10
Preheat overn to 350°

Noodles: Of course, you'll need spaghetti noodles. I sometimes use linguine. Break in half before adding to boiling pot.

Beef and Onion: The meat sauce starts with a mixture of ground beef and diced onion. You can also use Costco chicken meatballs, cut up.

Sauce: My cheat—a large jar 28 oz jar of meatless spaghetti sauce is the secret ingredient. *I like Raos brand.*

Salt: Seasoned salt enhances the overall flavor. Pepper and basil to your liking. Garlic, too, if that's a preference.

Black Olives: 1 large can, sliced

Cream of Mushroom Soup: 1 can

Mushrooms: ½ to 1 C canned sliced or fresh, if you would like to add.

2 Eggs: Eggs lend moisture and help hold the baked spaghetti together.

Cheeses: 2 C. You'll need Parmesan, mozzarella (maybe), cheddar, or mixed Mexican blend (my preference), and cottage cheeses. OK, you can add more.

Butter: 5 tablespoons of melted butter gives the dish extra richness.

continued

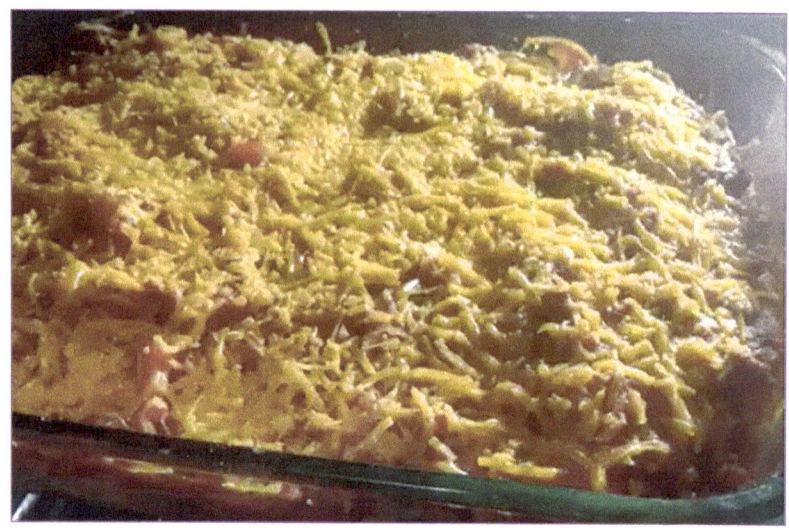

putting it all together

Boil and drain the spaghetti. Cook the beef and onion together, then drain off the excess oil. Add the sauce and salt and spices.

Whisk the eggs, cheeses, and butter in a separate bowl. Now, toss the spaghetti into this mixture.

In a large 11 x 15 (or two smaller ones), rub the sides with a little butter. The, layer the ingredients.

Cover with foil and bake for 50 minutes. Sprinkle with more of the cheddar type cheese for topping, then keep baking until the cheese is melted, bubbles. This is a BIG dish.

Judith's Friday Night Mexican Spaghetti Carbonara

One of my "open the pantry/fridge and what is here" concoctions. Yummers hit. AND, perfect for COMFORT food in Fall and Winter.

ingredients

Thin spaghetti (because I like it better than the thicker) (save ½ C of pasta water after cooking). *OK, if you forget to save … tap water will do.*

Bacon … at least 6 slices-you may want more

Garlic … I like lots, so I use 4-6 cloves, roughly chopped

1 can diced Ortega chilis

1 can diced tomatoes … *I had a bunch of fresh tomatoes, so boiled, skinned and cut up the first time I made this.*

1 can corn, drained

2-3 eggs *(I like 3)*

¾ C Parmesan cheese (or less if you want)

½ C Cotiga cheese *(OR any shredded you've got)*

Basil … *had it in the garden … why not?* (or some parsley for the topping finish)

Olive Oil … 2 T

Cilantro for topping, if you like

putting it all together

Start cooking the spaghetti

Prepare garlic bread while cooking the spaghetti … why not?

Cut bacon into smally pieces … cook

Open cans—chilis, tomatoes, corn—to have ready.

Then … the rest goes fast

continued

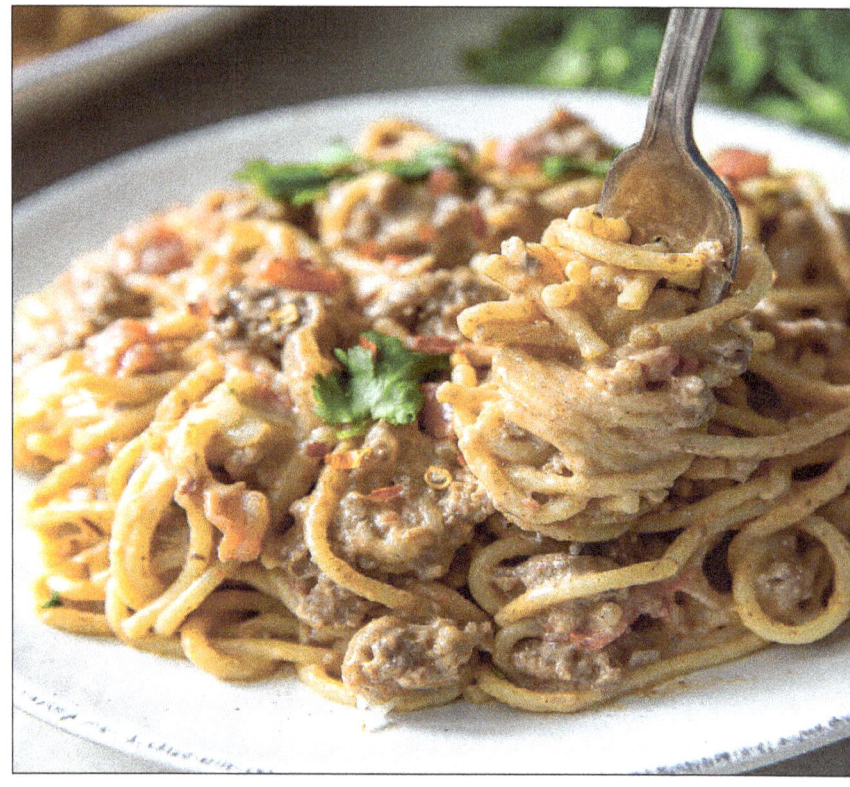

In large pan, add olive oil and chopped garlic. Saute.

Add diced chilis, tomatoes, corn, ¼ C of pasta water.

Cook water down.

Add in cooked bacon, then add in cooked spaghetti and toss together in pan. Add parsley, basil … whatever … in.

Cook until garlic is ready (this just takes a few minutes).

In separate bowl, whisk eggs, Parmesan cheese, other cheese, rest of pasta water (¼ C pasta water). Add to the large pan and mix until all is blended and hot throughout.

Forks ready … I serve in pasta bowls.

Judith's Mac and Cheese

When my kids are coming for a dinner gathering, they always want my Mac and Cheese. My "kids" range from a one-year-old great grandson to my oldest daughter who is 60. Sometimes it's the main course, sometimes a side. I always double the recipe. It's a take home favorite.

The difference from most mac and cheeses is the sauce. Mine is gooey … and it's the Velveeta cheese that brings the goo to life. After cooking the elbow macaroni noodles, you'll add the cheese sauce … and then baking it until it bubbles. Sometimes, I add diced Ortega chilis in the mix before baking for a bit of heat and French's Fried Onions on top for a little crunch.

Prep time: less than 30 minutes
Baking: 25-30 minutes.
ingredients

- 32 oz large Elbow macaroni
- 8 T butter – one stick
- 8 T flour
- 1 quart milk. *Sometimes I add half milk and half Half & Half*
- 16 oz Cheddar cheese-sharp
- 12 oz Velveeta cheese
- Salt, pepper, garlic salt or powder to taste, paprika
- French's Fried Onions
- *Options:* one small can Otega chilis, diced (for the adult version). If I'm making a large batch, I sometimes make half with the Ortega chilis, and half without.

Pre-heated oven 325°

continued

putting it all together
Cook Macaroni
Fill a large pot with water and bring to a boil. Add macaroni. Cook 8-11 minutes. Drain. Transfer to large , 9 x 13 baking dish. Any overflow, add to another baking dish.

Classic cheese sauce always begins with béchamel. That's the easy peasy white sauce made of butter, flour, milk, and a few seasonings. You will then add cheese a sharp cheddar to start that I grate from a block of cheese. Then add the Velveeta in chunks taken from half a block. Stir often to eliminate any lumps.

How to Make Cheese Sauce in 4 easy steps
You'll use 2 T butter and 2 T all-purpose flour for every 1 C of milk.

Grate your cheese. *Do not use pre-package grated.* It has a coating on it that prevents the cheese from sticking together. It can also produce a grainy sauce, not the smooth one you want.

To create the roux, melt the butter over a low heat. Add the flour and continue stirring to make a thick paste. When the flour is incorporated into the butter cook for a few minutes to activate the starch granules. The roux will thicken and turn slightly brown.

Gradually whisk in cold milk, stirring constantly as it comes together. *You can use fresh whole milk. Or I go to the pantry for a can of evaporated milk, sometimes two. I rarely have regular milk in my refrigerator and the almond milk I use for oatmeal won't work.*

Add in your seasonings: pepper, salt, maybe garlic salt or garlic power, paprika.

Add grated cheese to the white sauce a handful at a time. You want to melt it. Your goal is to have a smooth sauce.

Pour cheese sauce over the macaroni. *Be generous.* Add Ortega chilis for a little kick if you want. Add extra grated cheese on top. Bake until bubbles—around 25 minutes. Last five minutes, sprinkle French's Fried Onions on top.

Chile Rellenos Casserole

When I'm checking out a Mexican restaurant, I test it with a cheese enchilada and the chile relleno. It's gotta pass my taste buds. My cheat is a casserole version, with items that I always have in my pantry —evaporated milk, Ortega chiles, salsa, and flour. An easy peasy type of comfort food. Add a few tortilla chips and you are good to go. You could fix margaritas and/or have beer on hand.

Prep: 15 min. 9" x 13" baking dish with cooking spray
Serves 6 | Cook: 45 min.
ingredients

- 2 – 7 oz cans whole green Ortega chile peppers, drained
- 8 oz Monterey Jack cheese, shredded
- 8 oz Longhorn or Cheddar cheese, shredded
- 2 eggs, beaten
- 1 5 oz can evaporated milk
- 2 T all-purpose flour
- ½ C milk
- 1 8 oz can tomato sauce
  … for a little more kick, use salsa

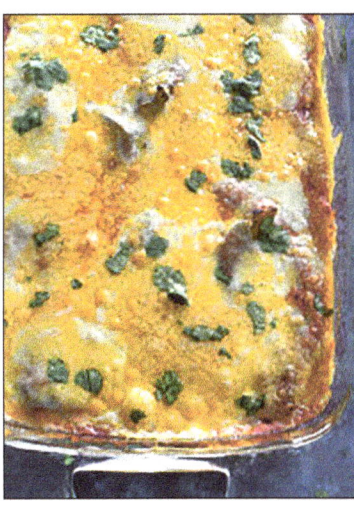

Preheat over to 350°F.

putting it all together
Lay half of the chilies evenly in bottom of baking dish. Sprinkle with half of the Jack and Cheddar cheeses, and cover with remaining chilies. In a bowl, mix together the eggs, milk, and flour, and pour over the top of the chilies.

Bake for 25 minutes. Remove from oven, pour tomato sauce evenly over the top, and continue baking another 15 minutes. Add more Jack and Cheddar cheeses.

Mexican Tortilla Festival

I had a holiday gathering of authors and needed a dig-in and tasty offering on a winter afternoon. It was so good, my guests devoured it before I could take a photo.

The major ingredients were already in my pantry, freezer and refrigerator—cheese, green onions, and lettuce. All I needed was fresh cilantro that I would serve as a side topping.

Pre-heated oven 375°
Bake at 30 minutes
ingredients

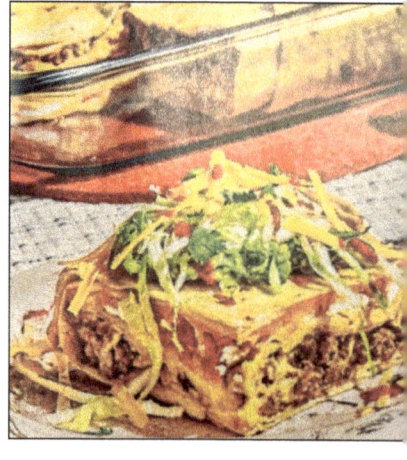

    2 C cheese, Mexican mix or cheddar, shredded

    1 onion, yellow or Maui

    green onions, one bunch, chopped

    1½ pounds ground beef

    1 (15 oz) nacho cheese sauce

    ½ C water

    4 T butter, melted

    1½ Taco mix packets

    2 cans (15 oz) cut or diced tomatoes, drained

    1 can olives, sliced

    8-12 oz sour cream

    cilantro bunch, torn

    12-15 large Tortillas, *fresh is better*

    10 Tostada shells, *premade or fry up corn tortillas in vegetable oil*

    Tortilla chips, crunched up

    Tortilla strips, *in the produce section of grocery store*

guacamole

iceberg lettuce shredded

Hot sauce, optional, for additional kick to taste

putting it all together
In a large skillet, cook ground beef, breaking any lumps up. Add onion until softened and meat has brown about 5 minutes. Add taco seasoning and water and cook a few more minutes. Remove from heat.

Get ready to make BIG layers.

Coat a 9x13 baking dish with melted butter. Line the bottom with four tortillas. Line the sides with tortillas with half of each tortilla overlapping the sides. Sprinkle cheese over tortillas. Add olives and tomatoes. Spread sour cream over the tomatoes.

Layer tostado shells over the sour cream, then spread nacho sauce. Add the beef mixture. If you want hot sauce, this is the time to sprinkle over the beef. Now, fold over the tortillas that are on the sides of your baking dish and fold them over the top of the dish. With the remaining melted butter, brush the tops. Don't be shy about pressing it all together with your hands.

Bake for about 30 minutes, until the top is golden brown. Let it rest for 5 to 10 minutes.

You are going to flip this, like an upside-down cake on a large platter. The bottom will become the top. Add shredded lettuce and green onions. I have a large bowl of guacamole for the quac lovers, cilantro, and tortilla strips for toppings.

Taco Pie

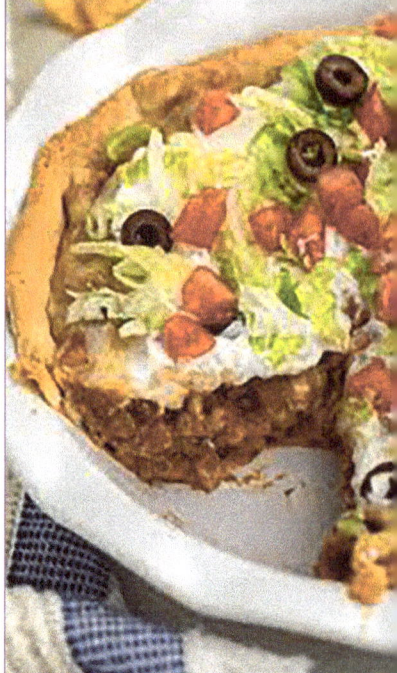

How about a variation of Taco Tuesday with a Taco Pie? I've always loved anything Mexican, so this is right up my alley for a super easy meal … or an appetizer for the gang.

Serves 8
Preheat oven to 350° F
ingredients

    1 8 oz package refrigerated crescent rolls

    1 pound ground beef

    1 oz package taco seasoning mix

    8 oz Mexican-style cheese blend, shredded

toppings

sour cream	green onions	olives	salsa
diced tomatoes	avocado	hot sauce	Fritos

putting it all together

Cover a round or square cake pan with the crescent dough flat on the bottom. Bake according to package directions.

Cook the beef until it is no longer pink.

Add the taco seasoning, stirring to combine.

When the crust is done baking, add the beef to the crust and then layer with the cheese.

Return to oven and bake until the cheese is melted, about 10 minutes.

Add your choice of toppings.

Cod Fritters with Mango Salsa

Back to my foodie group ... the dinner theme was Caribbean; I had my appetizer hat on. Usually, I will make three. Two of mine were the Fritters and a Mango Salsa for the add. I had never made fritters before. Delicious! All agreed a keeper—and some friends took leftovers and salsa home with them.

Prep: 25 min. | Cook: 15 min.
ingredients

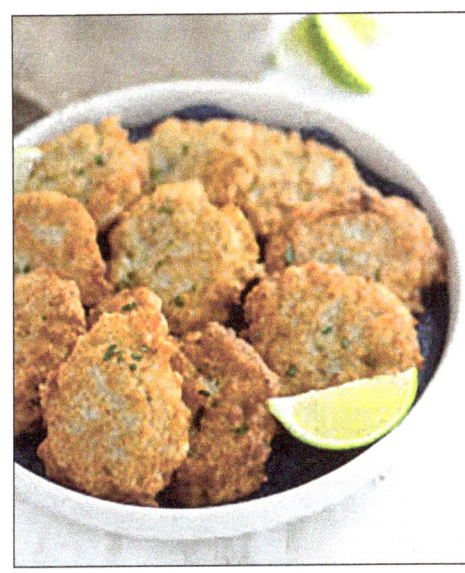

½ pound boneless salted cod or any firm-fleshed white fish

1 C all-purpose flour

2 tsp baking powder

1 tsp granulated garlic

1 tsp paprika

½ tsp sugar

1 medium onion, finely diced

2 Jalapeños, seeded and diced

2 T yellow or red bell pepper, minced

3 T parsley, minced

1 large egg

⅓ to ½ C milk or water

freshly grated pepper to taste

vegetable oil for frying (about 2 cups)

putting it all together
Must do ... Soak the cod in cold water overnight or for a few days (changing the water several times). Drain and shred by hand.

continued

Combine the dry ingredients: flour, baking powder, smoked paprika, granulated garlic, and sugar. Stir for about a minute, then add shredded cod, onion, Jalapeños, bell pepper, parsley, and egg. Then whisk these ingredients until well combined.

Now, gradually add milk, starting from about ⅓ C, until reaching the desired thickness.

Heat the oil until hot.

Adjust seasonings, frying up a small piece to do a taste test if necessary.

Carefully lower spoonfuls of the batter into the hot oil and fry for 3 to 4 minutes or until the fritters are crisp and golden brown. Do in batches.

Remove the cooked fritters from the pan with a slotted spoon and set aside on a paper-towel-lined plate to remove excess oil.

Mango Salsa

If you like fruit, a little sweetness with fish dishes, and dipping, my mango salsa is ideal as the fresh fruit becomes available. I always marvel at the size of the seeds these babies produce.

- ½ C cilantro, fresh
- 2 green onions, chopped
- 1 Jalapeño, seeded and diced
- 2 limes, squeezed
- 2 mangos, cut up
- 1 red bell pepper, diced
- Salt and pepper

putting it all together
Mix it all together, than CHILL before serving.

Shrimp with Corn Salad

I always think outdoors when I create and serve my Shrimp and Corn Salad. I'll have a tall glass of peach iced tea; John will have Sauvignon Blanc or a Chardonnay. This salad is perfect for lunch or dinner on our deck and just chilling out.

Serves 4 to 6

ingredients shrim

1 pound of shrimp, peeled and deveined

Chill for 30 min. Dry, sprinkle with chili powder (no salt needed)

Sear shrimp – no oil needed. Stop cooking when edges of veins are opaque.

ingredients corn

3 C of corn (about 4 ears or 3 C frozen)

1 red bell pepper, thinly sliced

1 C red onion

1 can black beans, drained and rinsed

1 avocado, sliced or in chunks

½ C cherry tomatoes, cut

2 T chopped fresh chives

2 T white wine vinegar

1 T olive oil

1 to 2 T lime juice

Lettuce, use your favorite

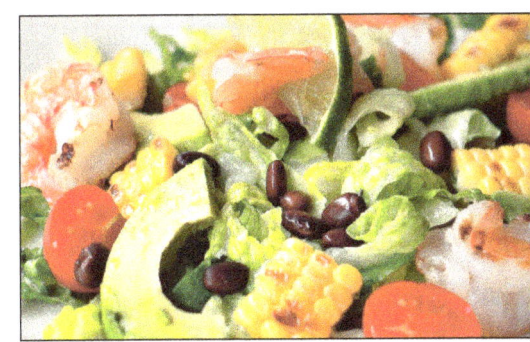

putting it all together

Boil or grill ears of corn or cook frozen per instructions.

Combine corn, bell pepper, and red onion. Saute for 5 minutes Transfer to bowl: add chives, vinegar, and oil. Add lime juice to taste.

Serve on a bed of your favorite lettuce with shrimp mixed in.
I always choose a romaine or iceberg lettuce for the crunch factor.

Judith's Ham Steaks and Cheesy Scalloped Potato Cheat

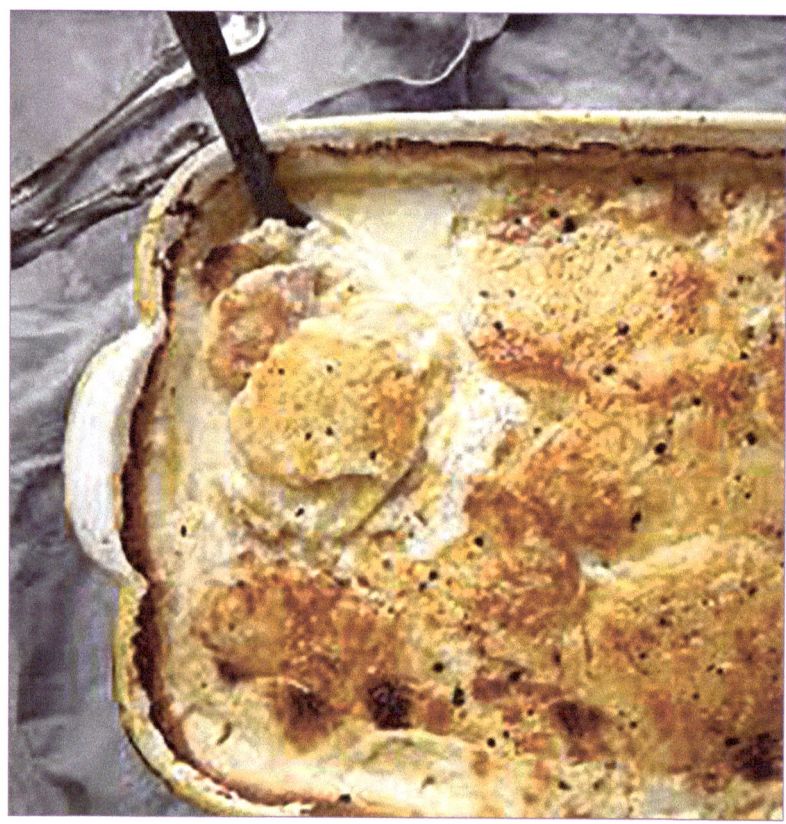

This is a delicious no-brainer ... four ingredients: ham, potatoes, cream, cheese. And choice of spices: salt and pepper, a bit of garlic salt, or lemon pepper.

Serves 6

to Costo you go

1 Kirkland, precooked, half ham in the Deli section of Costco or ham from your grocery.

1 package already prepared Baked Scalloped Potatoes *(use two if cooking for a crowd)*

½ C cream

salt and pepper, garlic salt, lemon pepper (all optional)

½ C cheddar cheese, grated

putting it all together

Cut ham into ½ inch slices. *I trim away the fat.*

Place in a 9" x 13" casserole dish. Top with baked scalloped potatoes. Pour cream over top for added moisture.

Sprinkle seasonings of choice on top, then sprinkle cheese on top of spices. Bake for 30 minutes or until bubbles.

Delicious. I always freeze servings for two or four for later. Asparagus or salad is a nice add.

Asparagus

Rinse stalks and trim ends.

In a small baking pan or cookie sheet with edges, place asparagus in a single layer. Sprinkle with 1 tablespoon olive oil, then ¼ cup Parmesan cheese. Toss to coat.

Add asparagus to same oven with Ham and Potatoes in the last 6-8 minutes of baking. *Yummers!*

Judith's Pork Loin Medallions

This was something I made when I discovered a pork tenderloin in my freezer. Quickly thawed, I just started adding simple ingredients from the fridge and pantry. The cream adds a yummy taste to the sauce along with the broth.

Pre-heated oven 375°
Bake no more than 30 minutes
ingredients

> 1 pork loin … cut into medallions of 1 to 1½ inch thick
>
> 1 can cream of mushroom soup
>
> Mushrooms sliced … your choice of type and how many. *I use at least 8.*
>
> 1 onion, diced. *I like the sweet yellow or Maui.*
>
> ¼ to ⅓ C capers
>
> 1 C half and half or heavy cream. *I prefer the heavy cream.*
>
> Broth—chicken or beef
> *I always have a large jar of Better than Bouillion® beef, chicken, and vegetable types in my refrigerator and pantry.*
>
> Pepper to taste
>
> Garlic salt to taste
>
> Parsley or basil as a garnish. *It's something I don't normally have in refrigerator and not necessary. With my summer basil, I always dry several bunches, then chop for later cooking, storing in a jar.*

putting it all together

½ can of soup with pepper/garlic salt in baking dish bottom. Add medallions, onions, mushrooms, capers, cream. Mix in, then rest of soup on top.

Bake. Add a favorite sourdough or French bread for sopping the juices OR a Jasmine rice on the side … and a salad.

If you want a bit of crunch … add French's Fried Onions on top last 5 minutes of baking.

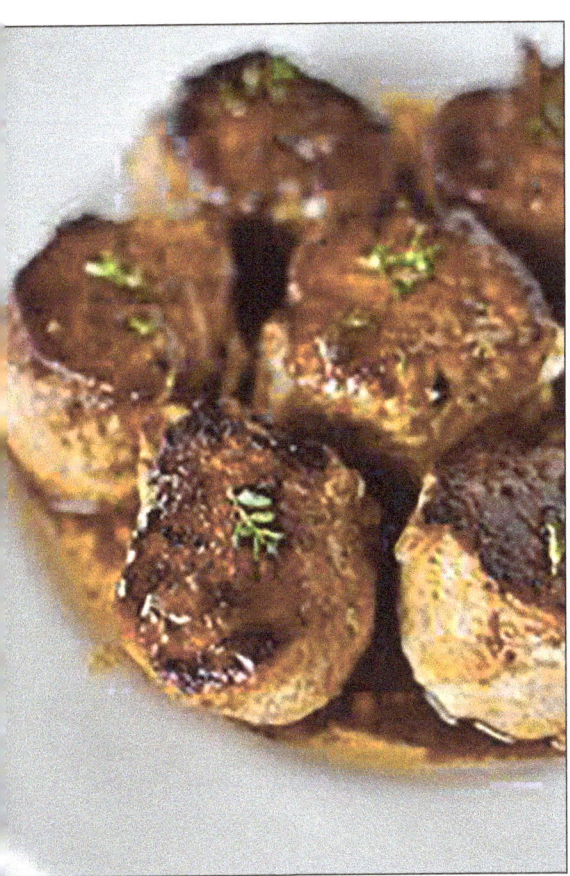

Oktoberfest Pork Tenderloin

This is definitely a Fall or Winter main dish. A side of rice welcomes the sauce that surrounds the tenderloins.

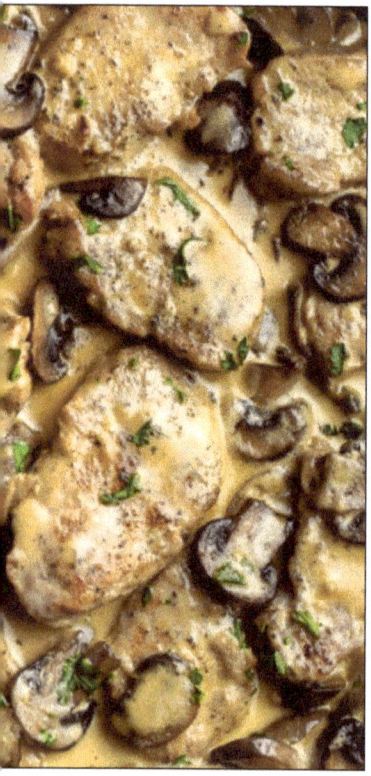

Serves 8
Pre-heated oven 375°
Including prep: total time is 45 min.
ingredients

8 pork tenderloins

8 strips of bacon

⅜ C brandy or cognac

⅜ C white wine

3 T beef bouillon granules

2 C heavy cream

3 T flour

mustard—dry or Poupon

½ pound mushrooms, sliced

putting it all together

Fry bacon until limp. Wrap around each butterflied tenderloin and secure with tooth pick. Drizzle brandy over meat, sprinkle with dry mustard or spread with Poupon mustard. Bake for 20 minutes.

Remove pork and skim grease from pan. Add wine and bouillon and deglaze over medium heat. Wisk together cream and flour and then whisk into drippings for about 4 minutes. Add the mushrooms and bake another 15 minutes in oven until sauce is thickened.

Chicken Swiss Cutlets with Avocados

We have this for holiday and birthday dinners ... it's a family and friends favorite. Warning: takes some prep time, especially with tenderizing the chicken cutlets. Once through it, it goes fairly fast.

Have two large baking dishes. You will be layering sauce with cutlets, then adding avocado and tomato slices on top along with Swiss cheese. Back to oven for five minutes and then serve. It's rich and filling.

Serves 8
Baking time 45 minutes
Preheat oven to 350°
ingredients

    4 chicken breasts

    ¼ C heated oil

    2 eggs, beaten

    1 C bread crumbs, herb or panko

    ½ tsp salt

    ½ tsp pepper

    1 tsp garlic powder

    ¼ C flour

    2½ C milk

    ½ C white wine

    3 T butter

    Mushrooms, sliced

    Swiss cheese slices

    2-3 avocados, sliced

    2 tomatoes, sliced

continued

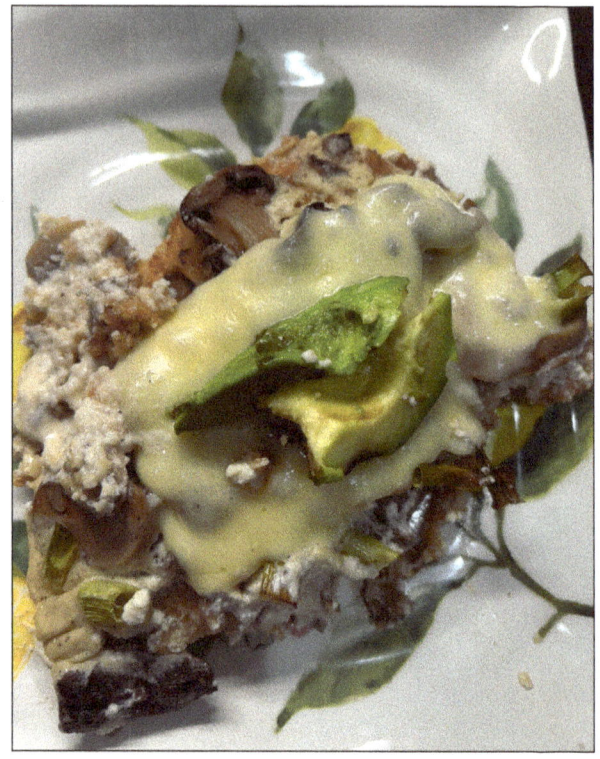

putting it all together

Cut the breasts in half lengthwise. Get out your meat mallet and tenderize and thin out each one.

Mix egg, spice mixture in bread crumbs and dip cutlets, browning for a few minutes on each side. Remove and do the rest.

Next, create your white sauce with flour, milk, wine, and butter. You will add half on the bottom of your baking dish. Layer the cutlets on top. Add sliced mushrooms and rest of white sauce.

Oven time: bake for about 45 minutes. Then, add Swiss cheese slices, avocados, and tomatoes as toppings. Bake another 5 minutes or until the cheese melts.

Serve with your sides.

Creamy Parmesan Chicken Cutlets

Chicken breasts are notorious for being thick and tasteless. No more. Most breasts can be sliced into three cutlets, cooked quickly to absorb the sauce you are cooking with. I usually purchase a six-pack of chicken breasts—to use in soups and salads. I decided to open and slice the six-pack into cutlets to freeze for salads and stir frys.

I had all the ingredients below in my pantry and refrigerator. In summer, I grow basil. In the winter, I've dried and stored the leaves in a glass jar.

Serves 6: two cutlets each
No oven time.
All cooked on stove top.
ingredients

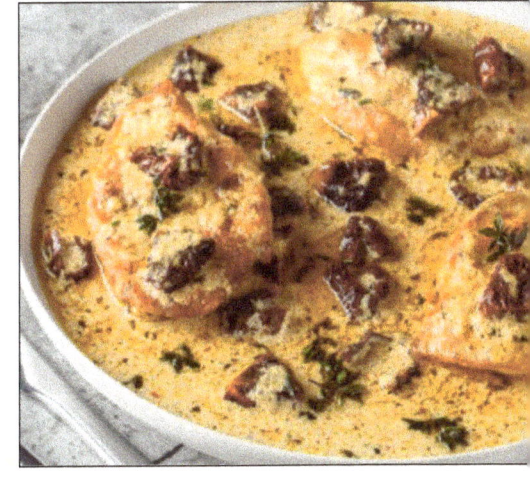

3 whole chicken breasts. *Costco usually has two or three whole breasts in a package*

Rice or Pasta, for serving

½ tsp salt and pepper

1 tsp chili flakes

1 T fresh basil chopped plus several leaves for garnish

3 T capers

6 T flour

2 T olive oil or avocado oil

2 T butter

4 cloves garlic, minced. *If I don't have fresh, I use course ground garlic powder*

1 C chicken broth
I love Better than Bouillon. Lots of flavors.

continued

1 C heavy cream

1 C milk or 1 can evaporated milk

1 to 2 C Parmesan cheese, freshly grated
½ C sundried tomatoes

1 can drained diced tomatoes

Mushrooms, sliced (optional)

putting it all together

With a sharp knife, slice each whole breast into three thinner cutlets. When you cut, your slices are parallel to your cutting board. These will deliver fork cutting tender pieces.

Season cutlets with salt and pepper, then dredge in flour.

In a large pan, add olive oil or avocado oil with butter. Cook for 3 minutes on each side until the cutlets are a light golden brown. Remove, cover, and set aside.

With a wooden spoon, sauté the fresh garlic in the pan for less than a minute. Add the chicken stock. Add in any bits of chicken left in the pan. Using medium low heat, add in cream, milk, and Parmesan cheese. Simmer a few minutes. Add in the chili flakes, chopped basil, capers, sundried tomatoes, and diced tomatoes. Add salt and pepper to taste. If I have mushrooms, I will add them to the mix.

Add cutlets back to the pan to cook a few more minutes. The sauce thickens as it simmers.

Serving … your choice. I've done it over a balsamic rice and pasta noodles.

Whatever you use, you want them ready, so cook at the same time as you are making main dish. Your favorite salad is a good add.

Judith's Plum-Glazed Cornish Hens

When I want to serve a festive dinner for a special occasion, Plum-Glazed Cornish Hens are a family-requested favorite.

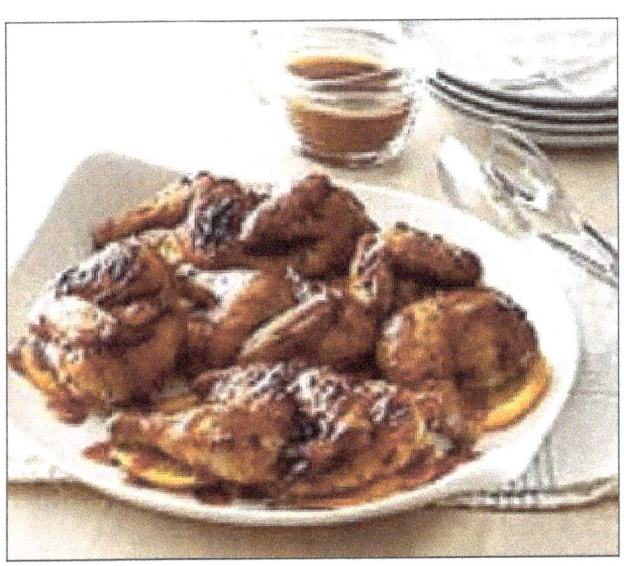

Serves 4 to 6
Pre-heated oven 350°
Prep: 25 minutes | Bake time 30-45 minutes

the hens

    3 large navel oranges, sliced – *leave rinds on and spread across a large baking dish.*

    3 Cornish game hens, split lengthwise and placed on top of sliced oranges. Spoon glaze sauce over hens.

glaze sauce

    ¼ tsp pepper

    2 cans (15 oz) plums, pitted, drained. *If you cant find plums, sub in 2 cans black cherries.*

    ½ C onion, finely chopped

    4 T butter

continued

¾ C thawed lemonade concentrate

⅓ C chili sauce

¼ C reduced-sodium soy sauce

1½ tsp prepared mustard *(I use Grey Poupon.)*

1 tsp ground ginger

½ tsp red pepper flakes

Worcestershire sauce

putting it all together

Open the 2 cans of plums: drain, pit, and set aside. You will add to the simmered ingredients below after done.

In a large pan, saute onion in butter until tender; stir in lemonade concentrate, chili sauce, soy sauce, mustard, ginger, Worcestershire sauce. Bring to a boil, then reduce heat; simmer uncovered for 15 minutes, stirring occasionally. Now, add the plums.

Remove 1 C of the glaze sauce to serve at the table for adds. Spoon remaining sauce over hens as they cook.

Bake 30-45 minutes longer depending on whether you halved the hens or bake whole or until a thermometer reads 165°, basting occasionally with pan drippings.

Warm the 1 C of remaining sauce for table use when all is ready.

Chocolate Zucchini Cake

Prep Time: 15 minutes plus for the draining of the zucchini
Pre heat oven 350°
Baking time 55 minutes
ingredients

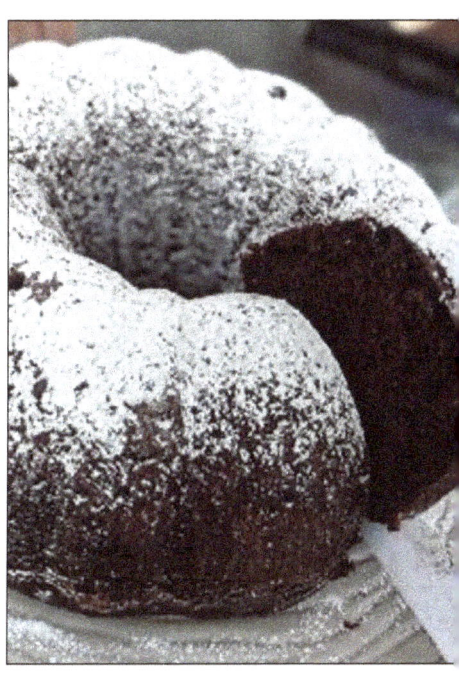

2 C all-purpose flour

¾ C unsweetened natural cocoa powder

2 tsp baking soda

½ tsp baking powder

1 tsp espresso powder

½ tsp salt

1 C vegetable oil

1 C granulated sugar

¾ C packed light or dark brown sugar

4 large eggs, at room temperature

⅓ C sour cream or plain yogurt, at room temperature

2 tsp pure vanilla extract

3 C shredded zucchini (3 medium).
Let sit in a strainer for an hour, then blot for excess water

1 C semi-sweet chocolate chips

Topping: chocolate or vanilla frosting.
Or my choice, just a sprinkling of powder sugar

continued

putting it all together

Make your cake: Whisk flour, cocoa powder, baking soda, baking powder, espresso powder and salt together in a large bowl. In another large bowl using a handheld or stand mixer fitted with a paddle or whisk attachment. Beat the oil, granulated sugar, brown sugar, eggs, sour cream, vanilla, and zucchini together until combined. Pour wet mixture into dry ingredients and beat on medium speed until completely combined. Hand stir in the chocolate chips. The batter will be thick.

Pour batter evenly into bundt pan. Bake for 55 minutes or until done. To test for doneness, insert a knife or toothpick into the center of the cake. If clean, it is done. Allow to cool completely on a wire rack. If you are adding frosting or powdered sugar, your cake must be completely cool.

Sheet Cake option: This batter will fit into a 9x13 pan. The bake time is at least 45 minutes-same oven temperature.

Cupcakes: Bake for 18-22 minutes or until a toothpick inserted in the center comes out clean with no wet batter. Same oven temperature. [High altitude adjustment: Bake time 25 minutes—until tooth pick or knife is clean.] Makes 24-30 cupcakes

Judith's Baked Pears

A perfect dessert and end of meal.

Serves 4
ingredients

- 2 T butter
- 2 T sugar
- 2 firm Bosc or Barlett pears, unpeeled, halved and cored
- ½ C heavy cream

Preheat oven to 400°

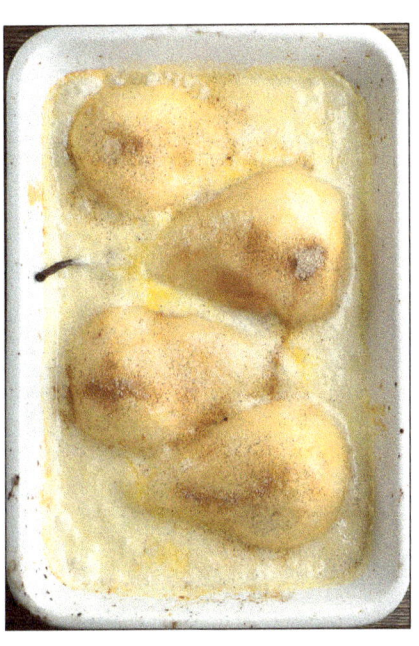

putting it all together
Butter a dish with 1 T butter, then sprinkle 1 T of sugar over the butter.

Place the pears, halved face down in the prepared dish. On top of the pears dot the remaining 1 T of butter and sprinkle with the other T of sugar.

Bake for 10 minutes. Pour the heavy cream over the pears and bake another 20 minutes.

The baking will soften pears so all you need is a spoon with each serving.

Serve warm ... *delish.*

Judith's Kahlua Cake

Preheat oven to 350°
Bake for 50-60 minutes
ingredients

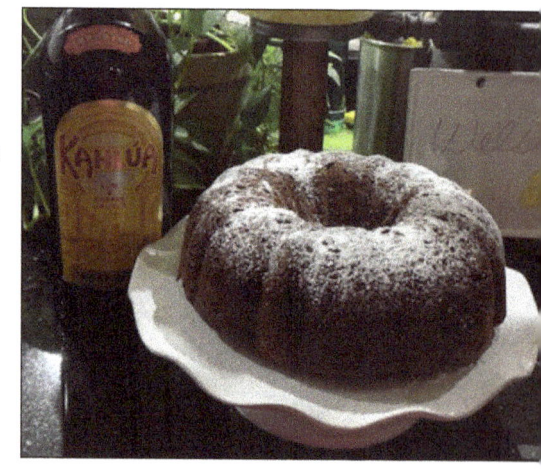

1 German Chocolate Cake mix with *pudding* in the mix

2 eggs

¾ C Kahlua

¼ C vegetable oil

2 C sour cream

6-12 oz of chocolate chips

1 T powdered sugar

1 pint Heavy whip cream

For high altitude ... add ¼ C flour

putting it all together

Grease bundt pan. In a large mixing bowl combine cake mix, eggs, Kahlua, vegetable oil, and sour cream until smooth. Fold in chocolate chips.

Bake for 50–60 minutes (knife should come out clean).

Cool in pan for 10 minutes. Flip onto large plate and sprinkle with powder sugar. *(I use a strainer.)*

Before serving, whip cream. Dollop each serving or scoop into a bowl for self-servers. *Decadent suggestion:* Add 1 ounce of Kahlua to whip cream or ice cream.

Tiramisu Made Easy

When I order dessert in an Italian restaurant, I always select Tiramisu. Sometimes it is served as a large dollop. And sometimes the perfect visual slice. At home, if I want a sweet dessert, I make something easy. Tiramisu can be easy peasy. It is rich and with hints of coffee, a kiss of almond, and, of course, CHOCOLATE!

I have lots of Tiramisu dishes and love to switch them up with the seasons—glass cups, elegant red crystal for Christmas, and a variety for summer-time deck eating. I also have dozens of mini glasses of different shapes and sizes—perfect for individual desserts.

This is a make-ahead dessert. There is no cooking.

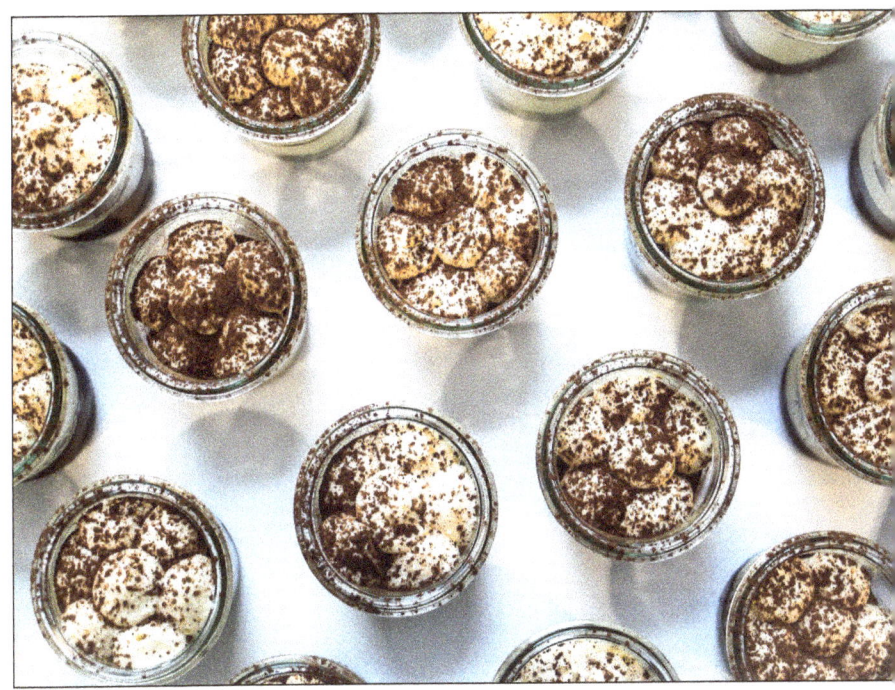

continued

Servings: 6 servings

Prep time is less than 15 minutes to refrigerator.

ingredients

    1 C heavy whipping cream

    ⅓ C sugar

    1½ tsp vanilla, *my favorite is from Mexico*

    1 C mascarpone cheese at room temperature

    3 T amaretto liquor

    2 C STRONG black coffee at room temperature, or use espresso if you have

    1 pack Ladyfingers, store bought

    Cocoa powder for dusting the top

    Option: add a few raspberries, or cut strawberries, or a kiss of orange zest as garnish

putting it all together

In a large bowl, whip together: whip cream, sugar, and vanilla until soft peaks form. Add mascarpone cheese, 1 T amaretto. Continue mixing until stiff peaks appear.

Combine coffee and the other 2 T of amaretto in a separate bowl. Quickly dip ladyfinger cookies into the liquid. *Do not soak—you are looking for the ladyfingers to pick up the flavors.*

If you are using small glasses, place the ladyfingers vertically along the outer edge leaving room to add filling down the center.

If you are using an 8 x 8 dish, add enough ladyfingers to cover the bottom of the dish. Add ½ of cream mixture on top of ladyfingers. Repeat with ladyfingers and remainder of cream mixture.

Using a sieve, dust the top(s) of dessert with cocoa powder. Refrigerate for 2 to 4 hours. Optional garnish: strawberries, raspberries, or orange zest.

Essentials for Judith's Kitchen

I have two pantries. One in the main kitchen that is used daily / weekly. The other is in the garage—backups and to "feed" into the kitchen when I need to resupply. Its companions are a refrigerator that is an overflow backup, especially when we have house guests or are entertaining, and a separate freezer.

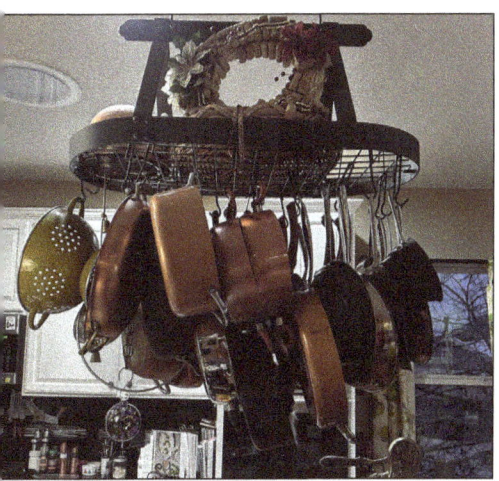

Most of my pots and pans are on a large rack hung from the ceiling. My knives are not put away. I have two magnetic racks that their blades attach to. And I have three containers that I keep extra "tasting/stirring" spoons in. Two are on each side of the stove top. One rests by a larger container full of wood spoons of all sizes and cooking utensils.

The third is on another counter I call the "drinks bar"—coffee, tea, and wine. All I need to do is reach and use.

My kitchen sink has two musts for me: an instant "hot" dispenser, perfect for a mug of tea AND a faucet that I can touch with a finger to turn on or off—sometimes a forearm if my hands are full of mixing up something.

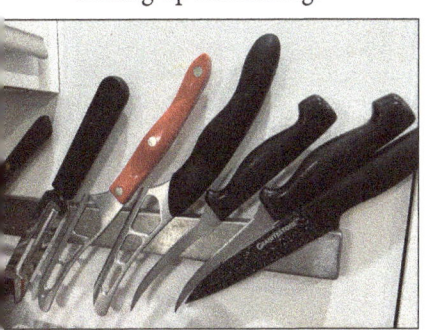
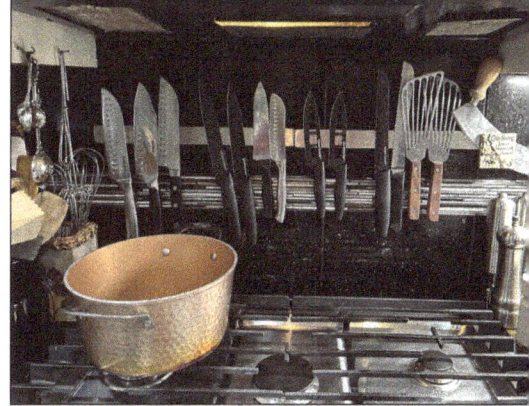

PANTRY

Albacore tuna, canned

Anchovies, tins

Artichoke hearts, canned

Avocado oil

Barbecue sauce

Beans: dried, misc

Black beans, canned

Capers, jarred

Chili sauce, Thai sweet, jarred

Chilis, Ortega diced, canned

Chocolate chips

Corn, canned

Cornmeal

Crackers, various

Garlic

Garlic powder

Honey, jarred and powder

Jellies and jams:
keep the ones you want … give away all others

Juices: apple and peach mango
Ketchup

Maple syrup, real

Marinara and fettucine sauces, Rao's, jarred

Mayonnaise

Milk, almond, boxed

Milk, evaporated

Milk, sweetened condensed

Mushrooms, canned

Mustard: Grey Poupon, variety

Oatmeal, regular and instant

Olive oil

Olives, canned

Olives, pimento-stuffed, black or kalamata

Onions: red and sweet yellow

Panko breadcrumbs

Pastas, assorted dried

Peanut butter, jarred and powder

Peppers, chipotle in adobo sauce

Peppers, jarred

Peppers, red roasted

Potatoes

Protein drinks, Premier

Rice (long grain, brown or Arborio).
Also 90-second rice from Uncle Ben

Salsa, jarred

Seasonings: herbs and spices—list out what you use.
My pantry door when open has a rack with eight shelves packed—salts, peppers, etc.

Shortening

Soup, Cream of mushroom, canned

Stocks and broths: Beyond Bouillion chicken, beef, vegetable

Teas: various. I always have British and Irish breakfast, Earl Grey, Peach, Mint, Ginger Peach, and Plum

Tomatoes, canned
(crushed, whole, diced, tomato paste or RO*TEL)

Vegetable oil

Vinegars: white distilled, white wine, apple cider, red wine, rice wine

BAKING INGREDIENTS

Baking powder

Baking soda

Flavored extracts

Flour, flour, all-purpose

Peppers: course, whole, lemon

Salts: Kosher, sea, whole

Spices: cinnamon, nutmeg, allspice and cloves

Sugar, brown

Sugar, Granulated

Sugar, powdered

Vanilla, *I use only Mexican*

COOKING

Blender

Breville counter stove. *I do have a gas stove top and double oven. This is an extra but is often the primary for small cooking/meals.*

Cookie sheets, multiple sizes. *I have 10*

Cutting boards, variety of sizes. *A personal favorite is The Pig. I made him in a woodshop during a summer 70 years ago and he's still in use!*

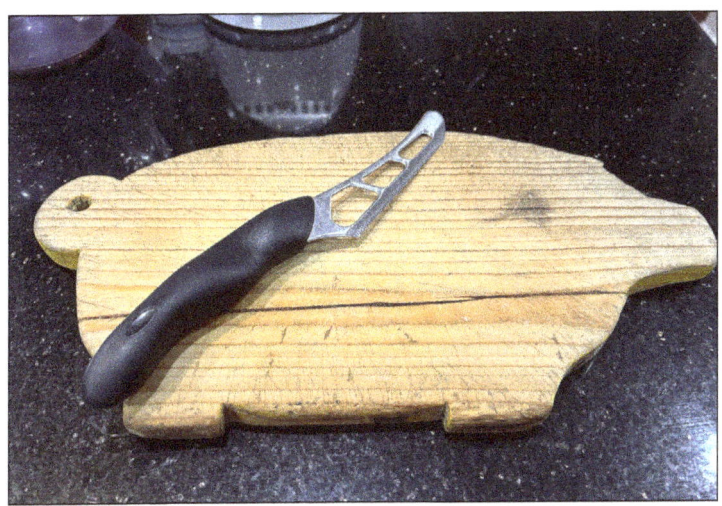

Fish spatula: I have three of them … most used

Hand mixer

Knives, variety of types. *Personal favorite is Cutco cheese and vegetable … the best!*

Knife Sharpener. *Always on the counter by the Breville stove stove I can grab quickly.*

Pans, frying and sauce, variety of sizes: round, square, large, small

Pots: several large for soups and large group meals

Roasting pans and racks

Slow cooker, large

FRIDGE

Almond milk

Bacon

Butter: salted and unsalted

Cheeses: cheddar, pepper jack, Havarti, Swiss

Condiments that are open: mayonnaise, mustards, capers, pickles, etc.

Corn tortillas

Cream cheese

Eggs

Fruit, fresh

Juices

Vegetables, fresh

FREEZER

Beef

Bread loaves

Chicken: breasts, wings, thighs

Chili

Fruits, frozen

Nuts: pecans and pine nuts

Pasta sauces

Pie crust

Sausage, breakfast

Shrimp, raw

Soups

Turkey, ground

Vegetables, frozen

In Gratitude ...

Every creative has others behind them, around them, underneath them, and sometimes looking over them ... to be lifted and encouraged to soar and stretch. Without them, my wings would be clipped.

My Literary Team
Rebecca Finkel
Peggie Ireland
Barb Wilson
Nick Zelinger

My Business Team
Meg Adverderada
Julie Bernard
Leah Dasalla
Leslie Hart

My Foodie Friends

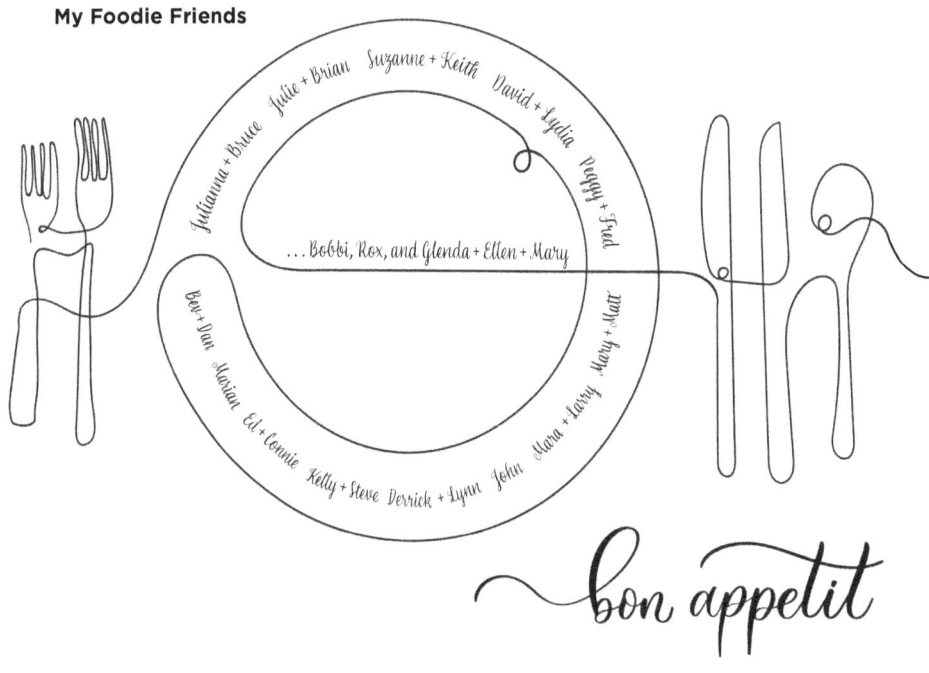

My Neighbor Friends
Ron & Melinda Adams
Al & Francie Bernier
Jill Taylor & Bob Cartmell
Kay Kelly
Rita & Frank Lucero

Gary & Janelle Mabie
Linda & Ken Nelson
Brock & Rita Norris
Glenn & Kathy Trice

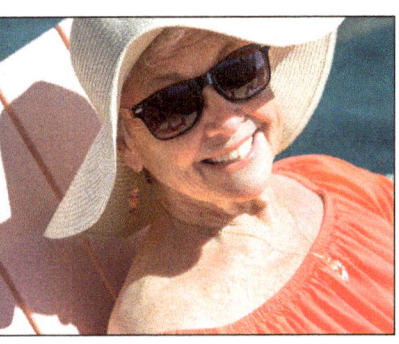

Dr. Judith Briles is the award-winning and bestselling author of 48 books and calls Colorado home. When she's not in the kitchen or in the garden, she's working with clients as The Book Shepherd, a book and publishing consulting and project management firm that works with authors at all stages of their book to create and publish a book they never regret! She's the founder of the first Authors' Hall of Fame exclusively dedicated to ensuring the legacy of authors connected in some way with Colorado.

Judith's books have been translated into 17 countries with over a million copies sold! They have been featured in over 1,500 radio and TV shows including repeat appearances on *CNN, CNBC,* and *Oprah*. She has worked with over 1,500 authors and created 500 plus bestsellers. Print publications include *Newsweek, People, Time, The Wall Street Journal* and … *The National Enquirer!*

Her publishing and writing titles include *The Author's Walk: Finding and Using Your Voice to Create Publishing Success, How to Avoid Book Publishing Blunders, Author YOU: Creating and Building Your Author and Book Platforms, How to Create Snappy Sassy Salty Success for Authors and Publishers, How to Create CrowdFunding Success for Authors & Writers,* and *How to Create a Million Dollar Speech.*

When God Says NO—Revealing the YES When Adversity and Loss Are Present is her personal memoir her reveals her multiple challenges to climb back when she was knocked down. To date, her books have earned more than 57 book awards.

Judith's historical fiction books are *The Secret Journey* and *The Secret Hamlet.* Book 3, *The Secret Rise,* will be published in spring 2025 and Book 4, *The Secret Awakening* in 2026.

Stay tuned for her next series, the *Silver Magnolias*. It celebrates the friendships and adventures of four women, starting with a weekend afternoon, a puzzle, and their favorite foods—recipes will be included within each story. And, she just may put together another recipe cookbook, *Appetizers with Judith*.

Join Judith's Circle for readers of her books for the latest book news: *www.JudithBrilesBooks.com*. Her publishing consulting is at *www.TheBookShepherd.com*.

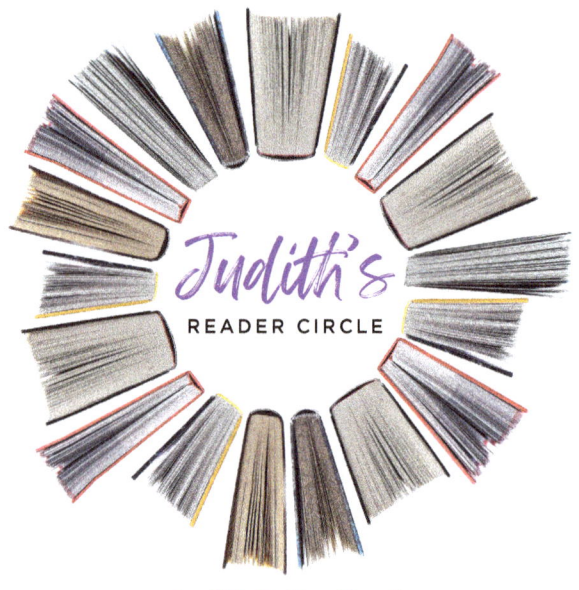

www.JudithBrilesBooks.com

www.ingramcontent.com/pod-product-compliance
Lightning Source LLC
Chambersburg PA
CBHW041147110526
44590CB00027B/4151